NURSING HISTORY REVIEW

S0-FQV-350

OFFICIAL JOURNAL OF THE
AMERICAN ASSOCIATION FOR THE HISTORY OF NURSING

ISSN 1062-8061
ISBN 978-0-8261-4366-2

AAHN
American Association for the
History of Nursing

2020–Volume 28

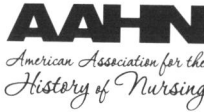

CONTENTS

SPRINGER PUBLISHING COMPANY

NEW YORK

The Role of Place in the History
of Nursing

Notes and Documents

Cover photo: American Red Cross Nurses. Reprinted with the permission of the Eleanor Crowder Bjoring Center for Nursing Historical Inquiry, University of Virginia School of Nursing.

Nursing History Review is published annually for the American Association for the History of Nursing (AAHN), Inc., by Springer Publishing Company, LLC, New York.

Business Office: All business correspondence, including subscriptions, renewals, advertising, and address changes, should be sent to Springer Publishing Company, LLC, 11 West 42nd Street, New York, NY 10036.

Editorial Office: Submissions and editorial correspondence should be directed to Arlene Keeling, Editor, *Nursing History Review*, University of Virginia School of Nursing, awk2z@ virginia.edu. See Guidelines for contributors on page XX for further details.

Members of the AAHN, Inc. (AAHN) receive *Nursing History Review* on payment of annual membership dues. Applications and other correspondence relating to AAHN membership should be directed to: Brian Riggs, Executive Director, AAHN, Inc., P.O. Box 7, Mullica Hill, NJ 08062. Phone: 609-519-9689. E-mail: aahn@aahn.org.

Subscription Rates (per Year): For institutions: Print, $239; Online, $179; Print & Online, $328. For individuals: Print, $144; Online, $108; Print & Online, $198. Outside the United States—for institutions: Print, $265; Online, $179; Print & Online, $355. For individuals: Print, $154; Online, $108; Print & Online, $208. Payment must be made in advance by check (in U. S. dollars drawn on a U.S. bank) or international money order, payable to Springer Publishing Company, LLC, or by MasterCard, Visa, or American Express.

Indexes/abstracts of articles appear in: CINAHL® print index & database, Current Contents/ Social & Behavioral Science, Social Sciences Citation Index, Research Alert, RNdex, Index Medicus/MEDLINE, History Abstracts, America; History and Life.

Postmaster: Send address change to Springer Publishing Company, LLC, 11 West 42nd Street, New York, NY 10036.

ISSN 1062-8061

ISBN 978-0-8261-4366-2

GUIDELINES FOR CONTRIBUTORS

The *Nursing History Review*, the official publication of the American Association for the History of Nursing, is a peer-reviewed journal, published annually. Original research manuscripts are welcomed in broad areas related to the history of nursing, health care, health policy, and society. The *Review* defines original research as that based on primary sources, that engage with relevant sources contextualizing events and arguments in the secondary historical literature, and in ways that allow the author to make novel interpretations. The *Review* prefers manuscripts of approximately 12,000 words, inclusive of endnotes.

The *Review* regularly publishes articles that later appear as chapters in books. Our publisher, Springer Publishing, holds copyright and the author and/or publisher must formally request permission to reprint the article at http://www.springerpub.com/permission-requests. The article must predate the publication of the book.

Conflicts of Interest

Authors must inform the editors of any institutional or organizational funding that has supported research related to the manuscript. This must also be indicated in the manuscript's acknowledgements.

Wellcome Trust

The publisher of the *Review* understands that research supported by the *Trust* are obligated to post final versions in a *Wellcome Trust* approved archive. Editors will continue to work with the *Trust's* requirements, *but authors must notify the editors upon submission of the manuscript.*

Preparing Your Manuscript

All authors should familiarize themselves with Springer Publishing Company Journals Policies and Statements (http://www.springerpub.com/journals-policies-and-statements/).

Manuscripts must be prepared using the guidelines specified in the most recent edition of the *Chicago Manual of Style*.

Manuscripts must be double-spaced and of letter-quality print. They must also use a type size of at least 12 characters per inch or 12 points. Please leave generous margins of at least one inch. All pages, including text, notes, and reference pages, must be numbered consecutively. All notes must be double-spaced and placed at the end of the manuscript as endnotes rather than footnotes.

Authors are responsible for securing permissions for all materials submitted. Authors will be asked to verify that they have secured written permission for publication of any interview or oral history data. If more than 500 words of text are quoted from a book, or more than 250 words from an article, or if a table or figure has been previously published, the manuscript must be accompanied by written permission from the copyright owner. Quoting from an unpublished thesis can be particularly challenging. If an author quotes more than five lines from such an unpublished thesis, he or she needs to provide a letter granting permission from either the author or the sponsoring institution.

Initial submissions of manuscripts must use *Editorial Manager* (http://www.editorialmanager.com/NHR/default.aspx). This system will ask for the relevant information about titles, authors, abstracts, key words, and manuscript. If applicable, acknowledgements can be included on your title page. *Editorial Manager* will also ask for a copyright agreement, with the printed notice that if a manuscript is rejected, copyright returns to the author.

Final versions of manuscripts accepted for publication will also be uploaded through *Editorial Manager*. Photographs or other figures accompanying the final manuscript must be attached in *Editorial Manager* as TIF files with resolutions of at least 600 dpi.

Author's Biographical Information

Manuscripts

The final version of an accepted manuscript should include a *brief* author biographical sketch at the end of the text of the manuscript with the author's name capitalized.

For example: PATRICIA D'ANTONIO is the Killebrew-Censits Term Professor, Chair of the Department of Family and Community Health, and Director of the

Barbara Barbara Bates Center for the Study of the History of Nursing at the University of Pennsylvania School of Nursing. She is the author of *American Nursing: A History of Knowledge, Authority and the Meaning of Work* (Baltimore: The Johns Hopkins University Press, 2010) and *Nursing with a Mission: Public Health in New York City* (New Brunswick: The Rutgers University Press, 2017).

[You may include an e-mail address here if you so choose.]

Book and Media Reviews

Book and media reviews will currently stay outside *Editorial Manager* as we adjust to the system. Your editors will give you instructions about how to format the introduction of your reviews. You should only give your name, credentials, and academic or organizational affiliation at the end.

Most correspondence about manuscripts will remain in *Editorial Manager*. Other correspondence can be sent to: Arlene Keeling (awk2z@virginia.edu). All correspondence regarding book or media reviews should be sent to your relevant editor.

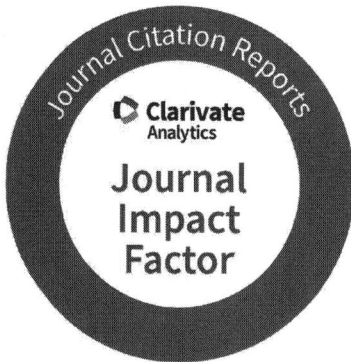

Journal Citation Reports
Clarivate Analytics
Journal Impact Factor

C|O|P|E

JM12778

EDITOR'S NOTES

Looking Back

I am not sure I know what to say. After eighteen wonderful years as editor of the *Nursing History Review*, I realized it was time to pass the torch to a new editor with a new vision. Any ambivalence I feel as I leave this position is thoroughly assuaged by the appointment by the Board of Dr. Arlene Keeling as the new editor. I have known Dr. Keeling for my entire professional life; and I count her a friend as well as a colleague. I can think of no one more able to carry the *Review* to its new mission and to sustain its role as the leading scholarly journal in the history of nursing and healthcare.

As Dr. Keeling well knows, it takes the proverbial village to ensure the prominence of *Review's* place. This is my chance to thank my village. I first acknowledge the enduring support of our editors at Springer Publishing: first James Costello, and now Adam Etkin. They have been unfailing in their support, advice, efforts to move the *Review* to prominence in our new online world, and lessons in the "nuts and bolts" of publication. My associate editor, Dr. Cynthia Connolly, has helped to extend the reach of the *Review,* and to work with authors who do not have their own village of support at their home institutions. And, of course, those who I consider the unsung heroes of the *Review:* our book review and media editors. Each year, they seek out the newest scholarship, find experts to judge its quality, and move reviews through to publication (tracking down the inevitable copyright releases that we must have). A sincere thank you to: Drs. Barbra Mann Wall, Brigid Lusk, Annmarie McAllister, Kylie Smith, Jean Whelan, and Winifred Connerton. Finally, an appreciative comment is due to the soul of the *Review:* our managing editors who keep our authors and us on track and on time: to Elizabeth Weiss, John Rutkowski, and Elisa Stroh.

One final thing I do know what to say. Although it may not often seem so, the history of nursing and healthcare has never been more vital to charting the courses our discipline and our healthcare system must take to meets its goals of access, quality, and affordability. If the articles that have appeared in

Nursing History Review 28 (2020): 12–13. A Publication of the American Association for the History of Nursing. Copyright © 2020 Springer Publishing Company.
http://dx.doi.org/10.1891/1062-8061.28.12

the *Review* have made some small contribution to that mission, I leave the editorship deeply gratified.

Disclosure. The author has no relevant financial interest or affiliations with any commercial interests related to the subjects discussed within this article.

Patricia D'Antonio
Barbara Bates Center for the Study of the History of Nursing
University of Pennsylvania School of Nursing
407 Claire Fagin Hall
418 Curie Boulevard
Philadelphia, PA 19104-4217

EDITOR'S NOTES

Looking Forward

First and foremost, I want to thank Pat for her 18 years of service to the organization and her dedication to making the *Nursing History Review* the top tiered journal for nursing and healthcare history that it is. Pat's ability to think analytically and communicate those thoughts succinctly is unsurpassed and is reflected in her editorial comments and the scope of the manuscripts that she has critiqued, edited, and published in the journal for almost two decades. A simple "thank you" seems hardly adequate. Pat, your legacy is a great one, and I welcome the challenge to continue to work with colleagues from around the world to document nursing and healthcare history from a diverse and inclusive perspective.

To that end, I will continue to (1) welcome the submission of the best scholarly manuscripts from the global community of historians researching nursing and healthcare history, (2) solicit manuscripts on methodology for a section on "Doing the Work of History," and (3) include the section on book and media reviews. In addition, I am initiating a section in the journal that is based on Dr. Barbra Wall's recent emphasis on "Hidden Nurses." It will be called: "Hidden in Plain Sight." So, with this edition, I am calling for papers related to minorities in nursing and healthcare history—those whose voices have been silenced in the past. And, since there is often less available data on these nurses, I welcome shorter manuscripts than the *Review's* guidelines currently call for, perhaps 10–15 pages.

As Pat has noted above, it does "take a village" to produce the journal, and I am looking forward to working closely with Drs. Anne Marie McAllister, Kylie Smith, and Winifred Connerton as they continue to serve as section editors. Thank you for your willingness to stay on! And before I go on: thank you Dr. Cynthia Connolly for your valuable contributions as Associate Editor. Your dedication to nursing and healthcare history is invaluable! As we look to the future, I am pleased to add two new colleagues to the editorial board: Dr. Christine Hallet, as Associate Editor, and Ms. Doris Rikkers as Editorial

Nursing History Review 28 (2020): 14–15. A Publication of the American Association for the History of Nursing. Copyright © 2020 Springer Publishing Company.
http://dx.doi.org/10.1891/1062-8061.28.14

Managerial Assistant. Dr. Hallet is currently Professor of Nursing History at the University of Huddersfield, Chair of the UK Association for the History of Nursing, and President of the European Association for the History of Nursing. Given her extensive experience as an author and editor, Dr. Hallet will bring valuable expertise to the position. Ms. Rikkers holds Masters and Bachelor's degrees from Calvin College in Grand Rapids, Michigan, and has worked as an independent editor for over 20 years. She is also my sister, and has facilitated the final stages of manuscript production for all of the books I have published. Her organizational skills and knowledge of Chicago Style are unsurpassed! Her experience as former Vice President of Zondervan Publishing allows her to serve as an expert liaison between the editorial board and Springer Publishing. Welcome to both of you!

As for the new process of manuscript submission, please send all manuscripts via email attachment to me at: awk2z@virginia.edu. Please include a cover letter, indicating the section of the journal to which you are submitting. I look forward to hearing from many of you!

Disclosure. The author has no relevant financial interest or affiliations with any commercial interests related to the subjects discussed within this article.

ARLENE W. KEELI
Professor Emerita
The University of Virginia School of Nursing
225 Jeanette Lancaster Way
Charlottesville, VA 22908

"Service is the Rent We Pay": The Complexity of Nurses' Claims to Their Place in Social Justice Movements

JULIE A. FAIRMAN
University of Pennsylvania

The relationship between service and social justice as it pertains to the health professions, and nursing in particular, is both simple and complex. Social justice and service are part of nursing's code of ethics, situating nursing's work with patients as inclusive and rights-based.[1] Service is tightly connected to social justice, and to what we do, how we are socialized, how our collective memory is determined, and perhaps most important, who we are as health professionals.

Nurses claim social justice as a critical part of nursing, and most of the time we can, but our claims are somewhat complicated. We all "tend to look to narrative threads from the past to the present in order to establish continuities in and meaning for ourselves"[2] and our professions. It is only by doing this, as David Hume noted, that "we have any notion of who we are, whether as individual entities or sociopolitical groups or nation-states."[3] We do have selective memories about our identities, but we may occasionally have to come to terms with aspects of the past, that on both a personal and public level, "we might rather be without."[4] The important point is how we use forgettable memories to create something different and better, for example, by using them

Nursing History Review 28 (2020): 16–30. A Publication of the American Association for the History of Nursing. Copyright © 2020 Springer Publishing Company.
http://dx.doi.org/10.1891/1062-8061.28.16

to understand the complexity of nursing's engagement in social justice rather than sweeping away and ignoring nurses' sometimes unethical behaviors.

In this article, which is a revision of the American Association of the History of Nursing keynote in San Diego, California in 2018, I will discuss service and its variations, social justice movements as complex entities and their connection to service, nurses as part of social justice movements, both as individuals and part of professional organizations, and the historical meaning of social justice for the profession. Underlying the narrative will be two broader historical questions: How can history inform us about nurses' place and identity as advocates for social justice? How can we come to terms with aspects of the past we would rather be without? Four historical examples, although none in detail, will be used to illustrate the complexity of nursing's claims to social justice: Lillian Wald, the Henry Street Settlement House and public health nursing; nurses work during the 1960s Civil Rights Movement; nurses in the Women's Health Movement; and the nurse practitioner (NP) movement.

Service, Social Justice, and Social Movements

Service in the context of the nursing profession can take on many historical meanings: Allegiance to a higher authority, work in exchange for something for example, quid pro quo, as a ceremony or ritual, or as a contribution to the common good in terms of tending to the welfare of others.[5] Religious women who nursed had an allegiance to a higher spiritual authority through their commitment to their order and to God.[6] Of course, the higher authority in nursing in the twentieth century could also have been an authoritative, unbending Director of Nursing! In the nursing profession, service also has a mixed history. Until the 1950s and 1960s, service sometimes had an historically negative frame of reference—the quid pro quo of student nurses' excessive hours staffing the wards in exchange for training, uniforms, and room and board. Hospitals used the rationale of service to justify student nurses as an unpaid labor force. Until that point, hospitals hired few graduate nurses because payment through traditional wage structures were not typical costs that hospitals assumed.[7] The third perspective, of service as a ritual, harkens to its religious connotations as well as the pinning and capping ceremonies that still exist in some schools today.

The fourth component of service, and perhaps most relevant to my argument of the connection between nursing's work, service and social justice movements, connects service as the contribution to the common good. The title of this article, "Service is the Rent We Pay . . ." is taken from a quote by

Shirley Anita St. Hill Chisholm.[8] The rest of the quote continues: ". . . for the privilege of living on this earth." Chisolm places service in the context of social justice, of the contribution to the common good and serving others, and is painted with religious and ethical connotations. In this way service implies efforts toward social justice, of being responsible for the welfare of others. Service, characterized in this way, should be part of nursing, as it underpins our legitimacy as caregivers, and our rhetorical stance as advocates.

Social justice and service are context and lens-dependent and can generate broader-scale social movements to accomplish a larger aim. Some nurses participated in social movements that resulted in death and destruction or marginalized certain groups of people in protection of tradition and the rights of particular populations, while others looked to broader missions of inclusion. No matter which social justice perspective, someone or some group will feel excluded or marginalized, and not all efforts to serve the common good, however it is defined at a particular time and place, are monolithic.

A recent example illustrate this lens-dependency. The Women's March on Washington in 2016, arose from a small group of women who coalesced through social media to millions across the world. The Right to Life march occurred in Washington a week later. Both events had common elements of women, protest and ideology, but different lenses. Both came from growing movements in response to social, ideological, moral, and cultural conflict. We find nurses in both the Women's March and the Right to Life March. Nurses in both of these movements believed their efforts were part of their service ethos and could improve conditions for the public. Both groups believed their protest supported social justice, but they targeted different ideological and cultural groups and resources.

The connection of service and social justice to social movements can be seen in the context of conflict over the "social use of common cultural values"[9] and the power to control resources to support a particular political (e.g., power, and not political party) frame of reference. Social movements arose in the eighteenth century, stimulated by structural changes associated with capitalism, industrialism, and perpetuated by new forms of communication (e.g., the spread of print). Social justice movements, a type if social movement, "are not neatly bounded entities, but are ongoing phenomena whose activity ebbs and flows, and whose parameters are largely defined by the observer."[10] They are not homogenous and they are not bound by time and place. Social justice movements tend to overlay onto social movements the concepts of rights-based allocation of economic resources from the perspective of human rights. They have the capacity for autonomous action, such as protest, both overt and covert. Historically the aims of social justice movements are at the least, three-fold, and are the same no matter the ideology or politics: the transformation of society through political and ideological conflict, class or social conflicts; changing the social structure; or to seek justice for particular groups such as workers, women, and other marginalized groups that are not always class-based conflicts.[11]

We tend to see social justice movements as any large-scale protest or social action that is visible and related to changing some piece of the social structure or seeking justice for various individuals or groups. That would be a fair way to think about them, especially in this time of modern social media, globalization, and pop-up protests where connections to common cultural values, such as equality, freedom, equity, and even nationalism may be quickly established. But I also argue we have seen social justice movements that from a liberal perspective were not always positive and were not just, but none the less can be considered movements tied to a particular perspective of justice. These movements had all the components of social justice movements: They were class-based, addressed the allocation of economic resources, and were focused on common cultural values that at that point in time were believed to have bettered society. The Nazi and Eugenics movement were, from particular perspectives, social justice movements for those who enjoined in their destructive aims. Although many in the profession might engage in collective denial and what sociologist Eviatar Zerubavel calls a "conspiracy of silence,"[12] nurses participated in both of these.

Nurses, both as individuals, and as part of organizations (although that is a complex history), have participated in social movements to improve conditions for themselves and the public, to put into place those things that support health in communities. But nurses have also supported other paradigms that are attempts to bolster nurses' status in health systems at the expense of other workers. Nurses' early twentieth century conflicts over the patient care territory with "professed" nurses or more recently, the debate over level of education needed to enter the profession are sometimes status proxies that cloud the impact of nurses' more altruistic claims of inclusion and of improving patient care through the use of better educated nurses.

Lillian Wald, the Henry Street Settlement, and Public Health

One of the most well-known examples of nurses participating or perhaps even creating social movements through service is Lillian Wald and her work at the Henry Street Settlement House in New York City. The settlement had a school, provided classes on childbearing, budgeting, hygiene, how tenants could get what they needed from landlords, and fire safety in an uncanny early focus on the social determinants of health and the culture of health.[13] Lillian Wald, as a young graduate nurse from the New York Training School for Nurses, began teaching a class in home nursing and hygiene to immigrant women in the neighborhood. She saw the squalor and the lack of resources to build healthy lives and prevent illness. Most of the people in the community could not afford care and illnesses that should have been treatable caused death or disability.[14] Her experiences helped frame Henry Street Settlement House as part of a reform movement bringing health and health services to communities with few resources.

Wald is an interesting example of a woman's individual actions coalescing into a national movement. With her friend, Mary Brewster, Lillian Wald established the Visiting Nurses Service and eventually public health nursing, which became a movement to keep people healthy in their communities. Public health nursing helped change the array of services nurses could provide to the poor, the sick, and to preserve the healthy. Even so, public health nurses were also known to be defenders of nationalist movements and disrespectful of cultural and religious habits of marginalized groups, such as immigrants and Native Americans. At times, nurses' own beliefs and values of appropriate behavior and health merged with efforts to Americanize their patients to create useful citizens rather than public charges.[15] Meshing these powerful impulses led to children's loss of ethnic and cultural identity, and in extreme examples, loss of parents and families.

Civil Rights

Nurses involvement in the Civil Rights Movement is also a very complex example. African American nurses like Mabel Staupers, a nationally known nurse leader, worked against strong opposition to integrate the Army Nurse Corp in World War II, part of what historian Jaqueline Dowd Hall calls "the long Civil Rights Movement."[16] Later, many nurses of all races participated during civil rights activities of the 1960s, although none of the volunteers experienced violence or discrimination on the same scale as black nurses in the south. Nurses in and out of the South worked for activist groups, including the Student Non-violent Coordinating Committee and the Medical Committee for Human Rights. They marched with Dr. Martin Luther King and cared for now Congressman John Lewis in 1965 after he was severely beaten by Southern law enforcement offices on the Edmund Pettis Bridge outside of Selma Alabama on Bloody Sunday. Nurses worked in rural communities across the south.

But, as nurses worked for voting rights and access to healthcare services for the poor and marginalized, many also worked to maintain segregation in nursing schools and hospitals. White nurses pushed black patients from white-only waiting rooms in clinics, and many worked without protest or concern in racially segregated hospitals or nurse training schools.[17]

While some American Nurses Association (ANA) leaders challenged social racialized stereotypes of nursing, local members of state nursing organizations in the south (and more subtly in the north) were denying membership to African American nurses even when they served their country in World War II. Some nursing organizations such as the National Organization for Public Health Nursing had always been integrated, and the National League for Nursing Education (NLNE), which required ANA membership, changed its rules in 1942 to no longer require it for admission. The NLNE's change reflected the shifting tide of both social and political pressure from their own membership to support integration. This was a direct challenge to the ANA to do something about the state organizations, which had become a public embarrassment.[18]

One of the reasons the state organizations could deny membership to African American nurses while the national organization debated integration is that the ANA reorganized in 1911. It became an organization of state associations rather than individual members. The North Carolina State Nurses Association did not end denial of membership to African American nurses until 1948, and was one of the last to do so (the American Medical Association did not require state association integration into the late 1960s, and then only reluctantly). Then, it was a matter of losing opportunities afforded by the ANA if the state associations did not integrate. The ability to participate in collective bargaining was a powerful driver to convince the white-only North Carolina State Nurses Association to admit African American nurses. In addition to these powerful economic incentives, the impetus for change came from a cadre of strong African American leaders like Mabel Staupers and Estelle Massey Riddle Osborne, the first elected African American Board member (1948–1952), as well as Shirley Titus, Executive Director of the California Nurses Association, who saw economic welfare as a powerful strategy to integrate the nursing profession.[19] Society and healthcare was changing. A shortage of nurses, the growth of hospitals, and changes in state and federal laws all contributed and provided the nest for social change to occur.[20]

Integration of nursing as a social movement was more than a racially-based movement for equality. As historians Chrissa Threat and Patricia D'Antonio have argued, integration was also a class-based and gendered movement. The combined connection of race, class, gender, and social status proved most powerful. Both African American and white nurses saw professionalization, particularly through more stringent education standards and rigid observance of strict hierarchies as a powerful way to raise the status of all nurses, except for those who were men. Nurses of both races also used their social status and class to protect nurses' income, work terrain, and authority in hospitals from other types of workers such as practical nurses and nursing aides.[21]

The Women's Health Movement

The Women's Health Movement of the 1960s and 1970s was another example of nurses' complicated engagement in social justice movements. The Boston Women's Health Collective began as a gathering of local women that grew to a large-scale movement. They developed the publication, *Our Bodies Ourselves* (first edition in 1970), that educated and shaped the health of millions of women.[22] Nurses and physicians were part of this movement—although they typically identified as women rather than health professionals—and worked to make the health system more accessible and less patronizing to women.

In the Feminist Women's Health Centers (FWHC) of the 1970s in Los Angeles that began with activist Carol Downer, NPs joined in the movement to provide greater accessibility to women's healthcare, and were valued as health-care professionals. The FWHCS promoted self-care most vigorously, but the "participants also saw nurse practitioners as allies in their struggle against medical paternalism, helping provide the services that weren't quite medical, but perhaps not legally provided by lay workers."[23] Feminist writer Sheryl Ruzak, in her book *The Women's Health Movement,* also makes the case for the politicized nurse. By utilizing NPs instead of physicians, feminist health centers demonstrated the effectiveness and public acceptance of nurses as normative providers.

Many women in the women's health movement went on to be nurses—there is no clear count but some women activists saw nursing as one way to engage in social justice to humanize women's health experience.[24]

On the other hand, nurses were sometimes seen as part of the patronizing and paternalistic medical system—and many times they were—aligning themselves with medical doctors and with the status of science. Historian Judith Leavitt described maternity nurses in the 30s and 40s as "strange young women on errands . . ." who did not talk to patients or help them when experiencing discomfort.[25] Nurses also participated as individuals in the forced sterilization policies of several states—not only in the south—and were part of the process of identifying patients in the community for sterilization and then getting them to the operating room for their procedures.[26] These were class and race-based issues that many nurses saw as the way forward to improve their communities from a very specific lens.

Social Movements from Other Lenses

Nurses were also involved in different social movements that were aimed at addressing class, political, and racial issues but in a very different way than for example, nurses supporting the Civil Rights movement. Nurses' involvement in the eugenics movement is one example. Nurses across the country believed in the eugenics movement, the dominant social and scientific paradigm till the early 70s, as a way to improve the nation. They learned about this paradigm directly and indirectly in their textbooks and from work in local public health organizations, which sometimes intertwined public health initiatives with "race betterment" strategies. For example, public health nurses participated in Better Baby and Fit Family Fairs, helping to highlight families with "normal" traits. Nurses also provided extensive education materials to the public to improve their health, using examples of "abnormal" children and families, typically caricatures of immigrant and black families to educate the public about the dangers of unhealthy habits.[27] Margaret Sanger, a nurse and strong supporter of eugenics, illustrates this complexity: she wanted to help immigrant women who were dying in childbirth, and she did, but she also believed strongly that women who were poor, immigrant, and feeble- minded should not bear children.[28]

During World War II, the National Socialist German Workers' Party was more than a political movement—it was a class-based, scientific and social movement. Many nurses and the major nursing organizations in Germany participated. Nurses had to belong to the party to practice. On the one hand many joined the party out of necessity in order to earn a living, but many participated in the atrocities of the Holocaust. In one example, the staff in euthanasia hospitals for mentally and physically challenged children and adults worked to meet the mission of cleansing the country of certain types of individuals. In contrast, individual nurses did resist by hiding patients, or fabricating records.[29]

Nurses were involved in medical experimentation. Although it is difficult to parse out how involved nurses were in cases where their behavior went beyond that of ethical standards at the time, Ken Kesey, author of *One Flew Over the Cuckoo's Nest,* reminds us of the explicit power nurses had over experimental subjects, and how they might have wielded it. He was a 24-year-old student at Stanford in 1960 when he volunteered to participate in a government-funded study of the effects of psychoactive drugs such as LSD. He describes the nurse (on which he based "Big Nurse" from the book): "Sometimes a nurse came by and checked on me . . . It was painful business . . . This was not a person you could allow yourself to be naked in front of."[30]

NPs Forming a Social Justice Movement

Perhaps one of the larger social movements within nursing itself is the NP movement. NPs challenged the reining social order of physicians as the only normative provider for everyone. This was a class and gender-based movement that confronted the cultural assumptions that underpinned medical care, while also challenging the distribution of healthcare resources for patients.

The role relied on nurses' tenacity and at times the courage of both nurses and physicians to break with traditional roles. The movement was sustained by the void of unmet healthcare services in primary care and by patients who offered support and engagement. As nurses moved into primary care, pediatrics and family practices, patients found them to be satisfactory and interested providers, followed their advice, and came to their clinics. Patients found NPs, both alone and in partnership with physicians, to be acceptable and even preferable alternatives to traditional solo medical care models. They then shared their experiences with NP care with their neighbors, friends, and families, helping to build community support from individual encounters.[31]

In 1965, University of Colorado public health nurse Loretta Ford, along with pediatrician Henry Silver, came together serendipitously to address the lack of pediatricians in rural Colorado and to formalize and strengthen the type of services public health and pediatric nurses had been providing to the poor in rural areas of the state.

But even earlier, nurse Barbara Resnik and physician Charles Lewis were also developing new models of care in the outpatient clinics at the University of Kansas. Nurses learned physical assessment and critical thinking to provide more continuous and sustainable care.[32] Ford saw the nursing practitioner role as a way to legitimize what she and her public health colleagues were already doing. "When it came right down to it," she noted, "we were making decisions . . . There was nobody else, and, the poor families . . . frankly expected you to make those kinds of decisions anyway."[33]

To meet these needs, Ford and Silver designed a post-baccalaureate curriculum that included courses rarely found in nursing schools at the time, but which provided stronger foundations to serve the patients nurses were already encountering. Students learned to better understand the underlying principles of healthy child care and patient education. Graduates of this program, armed with increased depth and breadth of their clinical knowledge, were called NPs.

For this movement to advance, patients had to believe NPs services could meet their needs and that they were safe. This was also a critical time (the 1960s-1980s) for nurses to expand their practices as patient loyalty to physicians was dipping in response to payment scandals and pharmaceutical misadventures. News about NPs traveled through broad coverage in the popular press, through newspapers and magazines of the 1970s and 1980s during a critical time of patient dissatisfaction. Some of the most widely circulated popular magazines such as *Look, Saturday Evening Post,* and *McCall's* published stories. *Ebony* discussed NPs in 1975 as a good profession to enter because of patient loyalty and rising salaries. Sources as diverse as the *The Wall Street Journal* and *Today's Health* referred to NPs as "'supernurses,'expressing perhaps surprise at nurses' competence as well as recognition of their ability to provide high quality services." A 1974 *Wall Street Journal* article noted that "supernurses worked in logging camps in Washington, and on remote Indian reservations . . . In Cambridge, Mass, 12 pediatric nurse practitioners handle 25,000 patient visits a year at five neighborhood health centers in the poor sections of the city."[34] By 1985, *The New York Times, The Washington Post,* and *The Wall Street Journal* reported on NPs in the main or health section and printed letters to the editor over 150 times.[35] All of these sources were accessible to the general public; they showed patient support and helped patients learn about NPs, which in turn supported the NP movement.[36]

Patients in areas without physicians took a leap of faith and found themselves joining the movement. There are examples from the early 1970s across the country, in Eustancia, New Mexico; Elk County, Kansas; and College Park, Maryland; of NPs taking over or opening practices abandoned by physicians who retired or moved on. The NPs might have communicated with physicians many miles away, or practiced on their own, providing care to people who needed services.[37]

Both individual physicians and the physician organizations recognized the value nurses brought to patients, and probably understood the power of the NP movement better than nurses did themselves. George Ferrar Jr., President of the Pennsylvania Medical Society in 1969 foreshadowed NPs' successful change of the healthcare system:

> Right now, how many of you are willing to supervise a satellite office, say 10 miles away—staffed by a registered nurse with additional training, who will be a screening practitioner, treat emergency cases, and other cases with nothing more than the availability of telephone advice from you? You say it will never happen? Such a person *will*

come into being with or without your cooperation and guidance, and if such a person comes into existence without our active direction, this health professional someday could become the *single greatest opposing force* that medical doctors have ever faced.[38]

And he was right! Nurses have become normative providers of healthcare in all places where people need services. Nurses have, in many instances, by virtue of their service to individuals, families, and communities become a powerful social force—a social movement—in shaping healthcare.

History and New Perspectives

The value of history is that it should help us seek newfound perspective from this complex story. In a recent *New York Times* opinion piece about the competing emotions and perspectives raised by Ken Burns and Lynn Novick's television documentary, *The Vietnam War*, historian Gregory Daddis suggests that historical perspective should help us question deeply held assumptions and "stimulate new conversations," and I am proposing the same, in this case, new conversations about nurses' engagement in social justice. These conversations should help us listen to and learn from "the multitude of voices across time and place, and perhaps most important, to the voices of those with whom we reflexively disagree." History helps us fathom "how competing motives drive humans to make difficult decisions, both good and bad."[39]

History, as a method and a perspective, provides a foundation for our critique of the assumptions that underpin modern practice, to continually question the instability of categories like race and gender, and to continue to explore and expose the ethical dilemmas in the history of health and medicine. At the end of the day, this narrative touches on the ethics of practice. Nurses, through our professional organizations, or as nurse Ieshia Evans showed us as she stood her ground against black-uniformed riot police in Baton Rouge as she protested police brutality in the fatal shooting of Alton Sterling (a 37-year-old black man killed by police),[40] as individuals, serve their community as best they can.

Service is the rent we pay as nurses and as health providers, as members of communities and as citizens—and our service *should* come from our historical presence with patients, and our involvement in social justice issues across time and place. We need to understand the value of our historical standpoint, and to question our rhetoric and our actions, as we continue to explore ethical dilemmas in health over time and into the future.

Notes

1. American Nurses Association, *Code of Ethics* (Silver Springs, MD: Author, 2015), https://www.nursingworld.org/practice-policy/nursing-excellence/ethics/. Accessed February 10, 2019.

2. Beverley Southgate, "Memories into Something New: Histories for the Future," *Rethinking History* 11, no. 2 (June 2007): 188, doi:10.1080/13642520701270229.

3. Southgate, Hume quote, 188.

4. Southgate, "Memories into Something New," 189.

5. "Service, n.1," in Michael Proffitt (Ed.,) *OED Online* (New York, NY: Oxford University Press, December 2018), http://proxy.library.upenn.edu:2817/view/Entry/176678?rskey=wXoKQM&result=1. The four components were chosen from a larger OED entry. These pertain particularly to my usage. Acess date is February 10, 2019.

6. Barbra Mann Wall, *American Catholic Hospitals: A Century of Changing Markets and Missions*, Critical Issues in Health and Medicine (New Brunswick, Canada: Rutgers University Press, 2011).

7. Julie Fairman and Joan E. Lynaugh, *Critical Care Nursing: A History* (Philadelphia, PA: University of Pennsylvania Press, 1998), 53–59. http://books.google.com/books?id=txDbAAAAMAAJ.

8. N.D. This quote is attributed to Chisholm, but the dates and source for example, place, context (as well as the actual text) are not identifiable. Mohammad Ali is noted to have said in *Time Magazine* in 1978, "Service to others is the rent we pay for your room here on earth." (https://www.infoplease.com/memorable-quotes-muhammad-ali). Shirley Anita St. Hill Chisholm was a United States Congresswoman representing New York's 12th District for seven terms from 1968 to 1983. She became the first African American woman elected to Congress. On January 23, 1972, she became the first African American candidate for President of the United States, winning 162 delegates that year. Marion Write Edelman, Founder and President of the Children's defense fund later elaborated similar perspectives: In her 1992 book, *A Measure of Our Success: A Letter to My Children and Yours* (Boston, MA: Beacon Press, 1992), 4–5, she wrote "Service is the rent we pay to be living. It is the very purpose of life and not something you do in your spare time."

9. Alain Touraine, "The Importance of Social Movements," *Social Movement Studies* 1 (April 2002): 90, doi:10.1080/14742830120118918. I have used his model of social movements to reflect upon social justice movements, as there are similar assumptions that pertain to the common good.

10. Doug McAdam, Sidney G. Tarrow, and Charles Tilly, *Dynamics of Contention, Cambridge Studies in Contentious Politics* (Cambridge and New York: Cambridge University Press, 2001), 11–12; See also Daniel P. L. Chong, *Freedom from Poverty: NGOs and Human Rights Praxis* (Philadelphia, PA: University of Pennsylvania Press, 2010), 71–103, http://www.jstor.org/stable/j.ctt3fhknw.7; Marco Giugni, Doug Mc-Adam , and Charles

Tilly, eds., "How Social Movements Matter: Past Research, Present Problems, Future Developments," in *How Social Movements Matter* (Minneapolis, MN: University of Minnesota Press, 1999), xx. accessed 2/14/19.

11. Alain Touraine, "The Importance of Social Movements," 91–92.

12. Eviatar Zerubavel, *The Elephant in the Room: Silence and Denial in Everyday Life*, issued as an Oxford Univ. Press paperback (New York: Oxford University Press, 2008), 1.

13. Karen Buhler-Wilkerson, "Bringing Care to the People: Lillian Wald's Legacy to Public Health Nursing," *American Journal of Public Health* 83, no. 12 (December 1993): 1778–86, doi:10.2105/AJPH.83.12.1778.

14. Sandra Lewenson and Donna M. Nickitas, "Nursing's History of Advocacy and Action ," in *Policy and Politics for Nurses and Other Health Professionals: Advocacy and Action*, ed. Donna M. Nickitas, Donna J. Midhaugh, and Veronica Feeg, 3rd ed. (Burlington, MA: Jones & Bartlett Learning, 2018), 3–24. Wald was active in many different efforts to remedy social ills. She helped establish the United State Children's Bureau and lobbied for years for the end of child labor laws so that all children to attend school. Wald advocated for education of the mentally ill. As an active campaigner for civil rights, Wald insisted that all Henry Street classes be racially integrated. In 1909, she was part of a group that went on to establish the NAACP

15. David Vecchioli et al., "'If You Knew the Conditions . . .' Health Care to Native Americans," *U.S. National Library of Medicine, History of Medicine (blog)*, August 2010, accessed February 23, 2019. https://www.nlm.nih.gov/exhibition/if_you_knew/ifyouknew_05.html; Jaqueline Fear-Segal, Susan D. Rose, eds., "Introduction," in *Carlisle Indian Industrial School: Indigenous History, Memories, and Reclamations* (Lincoln, NB: University of Nebraska Press, 2016), 3–14; Cynthia A. Connolly, *Saving Sickly Children: The Tuberculosis Preventorium in American Life, 1909–1970* (New Brunswick, NJ: Rutgers University Press, 2014).

16. Darlene Clark Hine, "Black Professionals and Race Consciousness: Origins of the Civil Rights Movement, 1890–1950," *Journal of American History* 89, no. 4 (March 1, 2003): 1279, doi:10.2307/3092543; Charissa J. Threat, *Nursing Civil Rights: Gender and Race in the Army Nurse Corps, Women, Gender, and Sexuality in American History* (Urbana, IL: University of Illinois Press, 2015); Jacquelyn Dowd Hall, "The Long Civil Rights Movement and the Political Uses of the Past," *Journal of American History* 91, no. 4 (March 1, 2005): 1233, doi:10.2307/3660172.

17. Julie A. Fairman, "We Went to Mississippi:' Nurses and Civil Rights Activism of the Mid-1960s Los Angeles, CA (2018)," in *The 2018 Fielding H. Garrison Lecture* (Unpublished; Los Angeles, CA: The American Association for the History of Medicine, 2018); Phoebe Pollitt, "Nurses in the Civil Rights Movement," *AJN The American Journal of Nursing* 116, no. 6 (2016): 50–57.

18. Darlene Clark Hine, *Black Women in White: Racial Conflict and Cooperation in the Nursing Profession, 1890–1950, Blacks in the Diaspora* (Bloomington: Indiana University Press, 1989), 183–85.

19. Patricia D'Antonio, *American Nursing: A History of Knowledge, Authority, and the Meaning of Work* (Baltimore: Johns Hopkins University Press, 2010), 146–57.

20. "Ada Forte," n.d. For example, in 1956 the Georgia National Assembly passed a law forbidding coeducation of blacks and whites, cutting off state funds if schools were integrated. This law was repealed in 1962, and Ada Forte, then Dean of Emory University's

School of Nursing enrolled the first African American students as MSN candidates shortly thereafter in 1963.

21. Eileen Boris and Jennifer Klein, *Caring for America: Home Health Workers in the Shadow of the Welfare State* (New York, NY: Oxford University Press, 2015), 30–32; Patricia D'Antonio, *American Nursing, See Chapter 6*; Charissa J. Threat, "'The Hands That Might Save Them': Gender, Race and the Politics of Nursing in the United States during the Second World War," *Gender & History* 24, no. 2 (2012): 456–74.

22. Kathy Davis, *The Making of Our Bodies Ourselves: How Feminism Travels Across Borders* (Durham, NC: Duke University Press, 2007). The first edition was printed by the Collective.

23. Julie Fairman et al., "Patients and the Rise of the Nurse-Practitioner Profession," in *Patients as Policy Actors*, ed. Hoffman Beatrix et al. (New Brunswick, NJ: Rutgers University Press, 2011), 224.

24. Sheryl Ruzak, *The Women's Health Movement* (New York: Praeger Publishers, 1978), 172. Ruzak's argument is about the politiziation of women's health care, including those who provided it.

25. Judith W. Leavitt, "'Strange Young Women on Errands': Obstetric Nursing Between Two Worlds," *Nursing History Review* 6, no. 1 (January 1998): 3–24, doi:10.1891/1062-8061.6.1.3.

26. Johanna Schoen, *Choice & Coercion: Birth Control, Sterilization, and Abortion in Public Health and Welfare, Gender and American Culture* (Chapel Hill: University of North Carolina Press, 2005).

27. Alexandra Minna Stern, "Making Better Babies: Public Health and Race Betterment in Indiana, 1920–1935," *American Journal of Public Health* 92, no. 5 (May 1, 2002): 742–52, doi:10.2105/AJPH.92.5.742; Martin S. Pernick, "Taking Better Baby Contests Seriously," *American Journal of Public Health* 92, no. 5 (May 2002): 707–8, doi:10.2105/AJPH.92.5.707.

28. Mary Zielgler, "Eugenic Feminism: Mental Hygiene, the Women's Movement, and the Campaign for Eugenic Legal Reform, 1900–1935," *Harvard Journal of Law & Gender* 31, no. 211 (2008): 211–35.

29. Susan Benedict and Jochen Kuhla, "Nurses' Participation in the Euthanasia Programs of Nazi Germany," *Western Journal of Nursing Research* 21, no. 2 (April 1999): 246–63, doi:10.1177/01939459922043749; Hilde Steppe, "Nursing in Nazi Germany," *Western Journal of Nursing Research* 14, no. 6 (December 1992): 744–53, doi:10.1177/019394599201400607.

30. Ken Kesey, *One Flew over the Cuckoo's Nest* (New York: Penguin Books, 2007), quote vii–viii.

31. Fairman, "Patients and the Rise of the Nurse-Practitioner Profession."

32. Julie Fairman, *Making Room in the Clinic: Nurse Practitioners and the Evolution of Modern Health Care, Critical Issues in Health and Medicine* (New Brunswick, NJ: Rutgers University Press, 2008).

33. Interview with Loretta Ford, by Julie Fairman, Gainesville, FLA, audio tape, January 19, 2006, ll. 309–312.

34. Fairman, "Patients and the Rise of the Nurse-Practitioner Profession," quote 220.

35. Claire Safran, "Their Patients Call Them Supernurses (July-August) (1975): 21–23, 51. Quote p. 22–23," *Today's Health Care*, August 1975, quotes 22–23; *New York Times, Washington Post, Wall Street Journal* data from ProQuest Historical newspaper data base.

36. This section is condenced from Fairman, "Patients and the Rise of the Nurse-Practitioner Profession," 215–30.

37. See for examples, Robert Oseasohn et al., "Rural Medical Care: Physician's Assistant Linked to an Urban Medical Center," *Journal of the American Medical Association* 218, no. 9 (November 29, 1971): 1417–19; Staff, "RN Reports on 1st Year in Practice(1886-Current File), July 6, 1972, (Accessed June 2, 2008)," *Los Angeles Times*, July 6, 1972, http://proxy.library.upenn.edu:2082/; Jennings Parrott, "Murphy' Needs a Doctor Who Likes to Travel," *Los Angeles Times*, June 13, 1974. Access 6/2/2008.

38. George E. Ferrar, Jr., "Keynote Address, 1960 Officers Conference, Pennsylvania Medical Society," *Pennsylvania Medicine*, June 1969, 9–10. Italics in original.

39. All quotes from Gregory Daddis, "What Not to Learn From Vietnam," *The New York Times*, September 29, 2017, Vietnam 67', https://www.nytimes.com/2017/09/29/opinion/ken-burns-vietnam-lessons.html.

40. Katie Reilly, "Watch Iconic Protester Ieshia Evans Get Arrested in Baton Rouge," *Time Inc, The Brief Newsletter* (blog), July 12, 2016. http://time.com/4403440/baton-rouge-protest-photo-ieshia-evans/.

Disclosure. The author has no relevant financial interest or affiliations with any commercial interests related to the subjects discussed within this article.

Julie A. Fairman, PhD, RN, FAAN
Nightingale Professor of Nursing in Honor of Nursing Veterans
Chair, Biobehavioral Health Sciences Department
School of Nursing
University of Pennsylvania
Philadelphia, PA

The American Red Cross "Mercy Ship" in the First World War: A Pivotal Experiment in Nursing-Centered Clinical Humanitarianism

MARIAN MOSER JONES
University of Maryland

Introduction

On September 12, 1914, a group of American Red Cross (ARC) nurses stood in their red-lined navy blue capes along the rails of an Atlantic Ocean liner as it steamed out of New York Harbor toward the Great War in Europe. "The white caps, the gray uniforms, the line of scarlet as the fresh sea wind blew back the active service capes, proclaimed their identity," wrote an ARC nursing leader who witnessed their departure.[1] These 126 nurses in their Red Cross uniforms, along with 30 physicians, made up the surgical teams aboard the ARC's "Mercy Ship," which provided aid to combatants on both sides of the conflict between 1914 and 1916. These teams established ARC war hospitals in Paignton, England; Pau, France; Kiev, Russia; Kosel and Gleiwitz, Germany; Budapest and Vienna, Austria-Hungary.[2] The ARC later sent additional teams of nurses and surgeons, whose activities lie beyond the scope of this article, to war hospitals in Belgrade and Gevgeli, Serbia, Yvetot, France, and La Panne, Belgium.[3] The hospital units focused on care of wounded combatants, in keeping with the Red Cross' mission to carry out its obligations under the original Geneva Conventions.[4] This effort, supported solely by private donations, reflected the country's own self-image as the sole remaining standard bearer for civilization and democracy amid Europe's rapid descent into the abyss of modern war.

This article examines the ARC Mercy Ship's work as an example of nursing-centered clinical humanitarianism and engaged neutrality in wartime. While scholars have debated whether the United States adhered to its stated

Nursing History Review 28 (2020): 31–62. A Publication of the American Association for the History of Nursing. Copyright © 2020 Springer Publishing Company.
http://dx.doi.org/10.1891/1062-8061.28.31

policy of neutrality in the early months of the war, the Mercy Ship's work provides hard evidence that the ARC—a quasi-governmental organization operating under the aegis of the War Department—made an earnest and sustained effort to do so in the face of serious obstacles.[5] The ARC effort communicated an unofficial but clear diplomatic message to the belligerent countries that American neutrality did not mean American apathy. At the same time, the article discusses how neutrality was sometimes more difficult for individual nurses and physicians, operating elbow-deep in the blood of one nation's wounded soldiers, to adhere to in daily practice than for the ARC to maintain as policy.

This article further argues that the work of the Mercy Ship nurses advanced US women's quest for full citizenship. At a time that women were campaigning for the right to vote in federal elections, and facing opponents who contended that full citizenship must be limited to men because they were the only ones capable of taking up arms to defend their country, the nurses demonstrated that women could withstand the rigors and dangers of work in a war zone.[6] When the United States entered the war in 1917, the Army, Navy, and Marines signed up their first large cohort of women for military service, and the Army sent over 10,600 nurses to serve near the Western Front.[7] The ARC and other voluntary organizations also sent thousands of volunteers to work in the war zone, while millions of US women participated in war-related activities on the "home front," from rolling bandages to paid work in munitions factories.[8] The Mercy Ship served as a successful test case for this later large-scale involvement of American women in the war effort, which then bolstered US women's claim to full, voting citizenship.[9]

Finally, this study illuminates the professional collaborations and conflicts that developed between and among US nurses and physicians in the war. While historical scholarship on World War I medicine is well developed, few scholars have examined the distinct ways that US nurses and physicians collaborated to provide care to wounded combatants.[10] Existing scholarship on World War I nursing folds US nurses into the larger pool of Allied professional nurses, with most attention going to British Empire nurses.[11] Yet while American nurses in this war, like their counterparts in Great Britain, Canada, Australia, New Zealand, and South Africa, were trained in a hospital-based educational method pioneered by British nurse Florence Nightingale in the 1860s, US nurse training had become Americanized through decades of development in US urban hospitals (few of which followed Nightingale's model of a hospital-based nursing school under autonomous female leadership).[12] American surgeons had also developed their own new techniques and systems before the war, such as blood transfusion to reduce surgical shock and new types of anesthesia.[13] US nurses and physicians had additionally developed distinct ways of working together in operating rooms. In 1908, leading Cleveland surgeon George Crile pioneered programs to train nurses to administer anesthesia—something that only physicians were permitted to do in Great Britain—and in the 1910s, US operating room nurses were being trained to perform surgical tasks.[14] Such collaborative, if unequal, working relationships in the operating room developed within a wider social context in which Victorian-era strictures on interactions between men and women were yielding to modern social norms favoring mixed-gender socializing and companionate marriage.[15] As this article will show, conflicts between Mercy Ship nurses and their supervisors, and between the nurses and doctors, reflected this uneasy transition between Victorian and modern gender norms. But these conflicts did not prevent the mission's success as an experiment in employing surgeon–nurse teams to meet wartime medical needs.

This article, based on analysis of nurses' unpublished diaries and correspondence, archival records, news reports, and published accounts by nurses and physicians, examines the political context in which the Mercy Ship launched, the substance of the work that its medical teams performed, and the gendered professional and personal relationships that developed during this work. While much medical history focuses primarily on physicians, this article foregrounds the experiences of nurses, whose work formed the core of this experiment in American clinical humanitarianism.

ARC Nursing and Medicine

For the ARC, the Mercy Ship became an opportunity to introduce its new nursing program to the nation and the world. The organization, founded in 1881 by Civil War volunteer Clara Barton, held official responsibility for fulfilling the US government's obligations under the Geneva Conventions to provide neutral trained medical volunteers to serve all wounded in military conflicts.[16] But during the Spanish–American war, Barton's ARC had sent only a handful of untrained volunteers to aid American troops and had mismanaged donations.[17] The organization subsequently underwent a reorganization in 1905.[18] At that time, the Japanese Red Cross attracted the attention of US military leaders for its system of effectively treating wounded combatants of both sides during the Russo–Japanese war, and for the participation of trained female nurses in this effort.[19] The new ARC, which became a quasi-governmental body under the War Department, was anxious to follow this example, and recruited a roster of nursing leaders to form a committee on nursing. In 1909, the committee enlisted Jane Arminda Delano, former superintendent of nurses at Bellevue Hospital in New York City and head of the Army Nurse Corps (ANC), to lead its new nursing program.[20]

From its inception, the ARC nursing committee set strict standards for enrolling ARC nurses. While Barton had accepted untrained volunteer "nurses," the committee agreed that the new ARC should only accept graduates of reputable hospital-based nursing schools.[21] These schools, based in major teaching hospitals, taught nurses to become the chief purveyors of modern hospital hygiene and care, as well as indispensable and obedient assistants to doctors. While the doctor alone held the power to diagnose and prescribe treatment, the hospital nurse carried out the treatments. Under the watchful supervision of the chief nurse, she administered medicine in rigidly scheduled rituals, bathed patients, applied antiseptic chemicals to injuries, and changed soiled bandages and bedsheets on a regular schedule, while being expected to maintain a caring, cheerful manner.[22] The committee also required a letter attesting to the nurses' good moral character, from a nursing superintendent or a nurse affiliated with one of the professional organizations for female nurses (a requirement that ensured exclusion of trained male nurses), and that any applicant be a registered nurse in any state that required registration.[23]

The ARC committee, and Delano in particular, considered character references to be as important as training credentials.[24] For decades, she and other nursing leaders had sought to stamp out lingering 19th-century stereotypes of nurses as untrained, unruly, sometimes drunk women, who did dirty work that no respectable woman would touch because it involved intimate contact with the bodies of male strangers.[25] To make nursing into a respectable profession, most nurse training schools strictly policed their students' behaviors in and out of the hospital: probationers who broke the rules were rarely given a second chance.[26] The ARC's requirements for graduation from a reputable training school and a character reference thus served to weed out anyone whose behavior allegedly did not meet these standards, and to protect the reputation of their fledgling nursing body.

The ARC committee also agreed to exclude African American nurses from enrollment, despite the existence of several well-established nurse training schools for African American women.[27] The Army Surgeon General's office had recommended this exclusion for the ostensible reason that it would be unable to find appropriate (racially segregated) quarters for these nurses in wartime. The nursing committee, whose members were all white, decided to follow this recommendation without protest or comment.[28]

The ARC's Bureau of Medical Service also dated from the period following the 1905 reorganization. In 1908, the ARC had hired a physician specializing in occupational health to head a new Bureau of First Aid, and conduct first aid demonstrations in factories, mines, and railroads.[29] In 1914, Dr. Robert U. Patterson, a physician with the US Army Medical Corps who had served in the Philippines and in Havana, was assigned to duty as head of this bureau.[30] Patterson expanded the bureau to become a bureau of Medical Service, but had little time to develop its activities and membership before the beginning of the World War.[31]

Organizing The Mercy Ship

When war in Europe broke out in August 1914, the ARC convened a joint emergency meeting of its International and War Relief boards in the stifling, paneled chambers of the War Department building. The attendees decided to charter a relief ship, and equip it with "hospital units" consisting of doctors, nurses, and other support personnel. They asked President Woodrow Wilson to make an appeal to the public to donate to the relief mission. The boards also convened a committee to charter the ship, which the press later dubbed the "Mercy Ship." Patterson headed a committee to recruit medical personnel and equip the boat with hospital supplies, while Delano agreed to call up the nurses from the ARC's roster of nearly 5,000 enrolled nurses.[32]

Immediately after the meeting, Delano contacted her friend Helen Scott Hay.[33] A native of Lanark, Illinois and graduate of Northwestern University, Hay had then graduated from the Illinois Training School for Nurses, the only hospital-based nursing school in Chicago organized on the Nightingale model, and had later served as its superintendent. Earlier in 1914, Delano had asked Hay to go to Bulgaria to establish a nurse training school in response to a request from the country's queen. The war put those plans on hold, and Delano now asked Hay to become director of nurses for the European war relief project. Hay agreed.[34]

The next day, Hay and Delano began selection of nurses for the relief mission. They favored nurses who could speak a European language, and only accepted those who had passed a medical exam and received or agreed to receive typhoid and smallpox vaccinations, while excluding nurses who were not white, native-born, or female.[35] All nurses except Hay were paid $60/week—lower than average US nurses' salaries—and had to sign a renewable 6-month contract while agreeing to go wherever the ARC sent them.[36] Still, the organization had little problem recruiting nurses for the mission.

The nursing leaders' exclusion of immigrant and male nurses reflected both logistical concerns and social prejudices. Their stated reason for excluding foreign-born applicants was the need for the nurses to be issued passports, but at the time all naturalized US citizens along with noncitizens who had declared an intent to become citizens could legally be issued US passports.[37] It is more likely that ARC leaders wanted to avoid diplomatic difficulties by excluding nurses who might be regarded as loyal to an enemy nation, or that their own prejudices or concern for alienating donors in an era of widespread anti-immigrant prejudice motivated these choices. In any case, they offered no extensive explanation for this exclusion, or for their exclusion of male or African American nurses from the Mercy Ship's units. While several reputable male nurse training schools existed, male nurses were not eligible for membership in nursing professional organizations, and these memberships served as leading qualifications for ARC nurse enrollment.[38] In an August 1914 letter to an ARC donor, Central Committee leader Mabel Boardman offered a justification: male nurses would not be accepted by the belligerent nations as they would be suspected as spies.[39]

Even with these restrictions, Hay and Delano found that some of the nurses they accepted for the mission had "distinctly European" surnames that might cause problems. Rather than sending these nurses home, they directed that all of the nurses on the Mercy Ship follow the European custom of being addressed only as "Sister" followed by their first name.[40] This practice contradicted US nursing leaders' previous efforts to establish American nursing as a modern profession, as it echoed centuries of practice in France, Russia, and other countries in which nursing duties were performed by women belonging religious orders who had little formal training. It also apparently astonished many of the nurses, but they agreed to abide by it.[41] "Now we *were* losing our identities; merging them into the common mold," Katherine Volk, a German-speaking Mercy Ship nurse from Lakeside Hospital in Cleveland, Ohio, wrote in her memoir.[42] The name "Sister" not only served this quasi-military function of diminishing individual differences among the nurses: by concealing nurses' ancestral ties to the belligerent nations it reinforced the organization's neutral stance.

Since the ARC had no roster of enrolled physicians, Patterson had to recruit them through placing advertisements in newspapers and contacting local ARC chapters and medical boards. Successful applicants were required to pass a physical exam equivalent to the US Army medical exam, or to provide documentation that they had recently passed a life insurance medical exam, and to show proof of vaccination from smallpox and typhoid or agree to be vaccinated on ship.[43] Each applicant was also required to provide a letter, preferably from a "surgeon of prominence" testifying to his "surgical ability and experience." The ARC agreed to pay $166/week for the assistant surgeons (the same as Hay's salary), and $250/week for the directors. The ARC received over 2,000 applications, and chose a group of white physicians from 19 states, who were all under age 45 and "actively engaged in the practice of surgery," or "serving internships on the surgical services of large hospitals."[44] The reasons for Patterson's exclusion of Black, immigrant, or female physicians may be similar to nursing leaders' reasons for excluding comparable groups of nurses, although US medical schools had over the prior decade largely restricted their student bodies to elite white men.[45]

The greatest problem for Patterson was recruiting capable directors for each unit. These positions required senior physicians "of administrative ability and also good character, and good professional ability, who are also so situated that they are able to leave their regular practice for any length of time,"—a nearly impossible requirement, according to ARC leader Mabel Boardman.[46] Many married physicians with children were hesitant to leave their families (and the practices that supported them) for extended periods of time.[47] No such problem existed with the nurses, as the US nursing profession was restricted to single women and widows, and most nurses were employed by hospitals or engaged in private-duty nursing, and could simply decline assignments, ask for unpaid leave from a superintendent who was herself likely an ARC-enrolled nurse, and get a new job when they returned. These differences between the doctors and nurses in the structure of professional employment not only resulted in the recruitment of some physicians of questionable abilities and reputations, it primed the units for interpersonal conflicts. Many of the senior physicians, accustomed to exercising sole authority as private practitioners or holding high positions in teaching hospitals, balked at sharing management of hospital personnel with chief nurses, even though Delano had given each unit's supervising nurse managerial authority over the unit's other nurses.[48] Additionally, the Mercy Ship's medical staff was populated with many single physicians seeking marriage and others running away from unhappy marriages and/or looking for romantic adventures. While some nurses developed friendships with the doctors and a few married physicians on the mission, others found themselves the targets of unwelcome advances.

On Board

Once the ARC had recruited doctors and nurses, it operated in a quasi-military manner to prepare these teams for service overseas. Each selected nurse received a telegram ordering her to pack one suitcase with a month or 6 weeks' clothing and supplies, and depart for New York within 48 hours.[49] Upon arrival in

New York, nurses and physicians reported to a docked steamship at the 96th Street pier and received their uniforms as well as cabin assignments.[50] The personnel were divided up into 10 units, most consisting of 12 nurses including a supervising nurse, and three or four physicians including a director. The ARC generally assigned nurses from the same local area and graduates of the same hospital training school to the same unit, along with doctors from this local area or hospital, believing that this familiarity would help them work well together.[51]

Ahead of their departure, Jacob Schiff, a philanthropist and Secretary of the New York City ARC chapter, withdrew $8,000 in various belligerent nations' gold currencies from the US. Treasury to distribute to the nurses as the first month's salary.[52] Even though the mission was neutral, Schiff, a financier of German Jewish background, actively supported the Germans as potential liberators of the Jewish people from oppressive Russian rule. Schiff later would unite Jewish aid groups to form a Jewish Joint Distribution committee to aid Jews displaced by the war.[53] Schiff's activities contrasted with those of many elite Anglo-Americans who had close ties to Britain or to the large American expatriate community in Paris, and who founded aid organizations such as the American Fund for French Wounded or war hospitals in England.[54] In its effort to remain neutral, the ARC between 1914 and 1917 coordinated its work both with groups of Americans who favored the Central Powers and those who supported Britain, France, or Russia.

On board, the units began training for war medicine. Such training mostly reinforced the hierarchical relationship between the surgeons and nurses. The physicians, however inexperienced, offered the nurses daily lectures on emergency surgery; the use of military surgical equipment; the treatment of contagious diseases; anatomy; the nervous system; public hygiene in military camps; and the metric system, which was used in most European hospitals. Under the physicians' supervision, the nurses practiced techniques for bandaging the wounded, and both doctors and nurses learned French, Russian, and German.[55]

The nurses' on-board training also included moral instruction. Every evening, Hay led the nurses in Bible readings and hymns.[56] While not all nurses shared Hay's Protestant faith, none openly protested this required ritual.[57] However, some were not happy about it: Lucy Minnegerode, supervising nurse of a Kiev unit, caught one nurse "reading a magazine during an interval in the prayers" on the first night, and resolved to speak to her. Another asked Minnegerode to be excused from prayer but did not give a reason.[58] Then, before the ship departed, Minnegerode noted in her diary, Delano came on board and told the nurses that "she wished no card playing or dancing done on the ship as we were to prepare ourselves for a very serious mission." Delano warned the nurses that they were under "observation," that "all misconduct would be noted and reported," and that "no second chances were given."[59]

While some Mercy Ship nurses grated at these restrictions, they were likely accustomed to such militaristic moralism from their superiors. In a 1906 *American Journal of Nursing* article, Charlotte Perry, superintendent of a hospital in Utica, New York, wrote about the "military discipline" that should prevail in nurse training schools. "Just as in the army, there are Generals, Majors, captains, etc.," in the hospital, there are chief nurses, she stated. Moreover, she emphasized that obedience to one's superior was a shared obligation of all nurses.[60] Student nurses were also trained to anticipate the every professional need of the physicians and chief nurse with whom they worked.[61] Their training additionally included restrictions on socializing with men inside or outside the hospital, and the expectation of chastity while in nursing service. Women who broke these rules or broke down under the strain of their training schedule were expelled from nurse training schools.[62] Physicians' training, by contrast, focused on the cultivation of expert judgment and preparation for the assumption of medical authority.[63]

Such conflicts between nursing and medical cultures soon became apparent on board the Mercy Ship. The physicians, led by the crew of retired Naval officers, drank in the evenings, then marched around the deck singing, sometimes grabbing any available nurse by the arm to engage her in the merriment.[64] While many of the physicians treated the nurses with respect and friendliness, others did not. In an instructional lecture, for example, Dr. William Magill, director of one of the two units being sent to Kiev "called Florence Nightingale a great hand holder and classed women with idiots," Mary Frederika Farley, a supervising nurse with the same unit, noted in her diary. Meanwhile, Commander E.H. Delaney, a retired Naval officer who was serving as the ship's engineer, announced that evening that he "expected at least one marriage from every unit" and led the doctors in bawdy songs, Farley noted.[65] A few days later, Farley added that a "Dr. McG" (likely Dr. Magill) "gave a lecture on obstetrics which was brutal and very personal, all for the entire amusement of the rest of the people on deck."[66] Magill, a prominent New York City physician and former director of New York State's Hygienic Laboratory, would later incur the wrath of his colleagues through his scandalous behavior, and be relieved of his duties by Patterson.[67]

When some physicians made physical advances on the nurses, the nurses were burdened with the responsibility to discern how to refuse these advances while preserving a cordial working relationship with the physicians. Volk described in her memoir how one of the physicians in her unit took a romantic interest in her the week before the ship sailed and convinced her to accompany him, alone, to Chinatown and the Metropolitan Museum of Art. When Volk continued to casually socialize with the doctor, Hay confronted her for "promenading on deck" with him. The 31-year-old nurse soon realized that she would be sent home if she did not maintain a proper distance from the doctor, and began avoiding him. The physician took this as a personal rejection and became angry with Volk. Volk had to work with this physician in a wartime operating room throughout her 6 months of service in Budapest, and she sometimes reported that he acted in a "disturbing" or cruel manner toward her.[68] When she became sick, another physician in the unit paid a visit to her and tried to kiss her. She slapped him, causing an uproar in the unit.[69]

The incipient social tensions between unit personnel were fueled by a diplomatic snag that caused a week's delay in the Mercy Ship's departure. Having been unable to secure an American ship for the voyage, the ARC accepted an offer of a ship from the German Hamburg-American line. The problem lay with its German crew.[70] The ship's first destinations were an English port, followed by a French port, and both countries indicated they would turn away any ship with a German crew. So Captain Armisted Rust, the retired Naval officer at the ship's helm, traveled to Washington to ask British and French diplomats' permission to dock in their harbors. When both countries refused to grant permission, the ARC had no choice but to recruit a new crew comprised entirely of Americans.[71] The ship's original crew members meanwhile objected to being thrown off of the boat, as most insisted that they had signed up for 60-day contracts. When the ship finally left port on September 12, several among the original German crew members stowed away—and were later discovered.[72] Upon docking in England, the crew found that the pumping engines—to be deployed in case the ship should spring a leak—had been sabotaged, likely by disgruntled German crew members. Fortunately for the passengers, the ship had not needed these engines during the passage.[73]

The delay in departure ultimately benefitted the ARC, which had initially struggled to raise funds for its war relief effort. When ARC leaders secured the ship, they had received permission from international shipping authorities to paint the ship white with a red stripe around the hull, place a large electric red cross on the deck, and fly Red Cross and American flags from the mast. The red and white Mercy Ship, while docked in New York Harbor, created a publicity storm.[74] During the conflicts over the crew, members of the public were invited on board for tours (prompting Minnegerode to complain in her diary, "They looked at the nurses, peeping in at windows, as if we were a menagerie . . ."[75]). Newspapers published photo spreads of the Mercy Ship and its nurses, causing donations to reach the hundred-thousand-dollar mark. "This act proved to be the magic lever needed to open America's storehouse of gold," wrote one reporter.[76] The ARC could now afford to purchase medical supplies. When the ship departed, it carried in its hull 4,000 pounds (1,814 kg) of cotton; 250,000 meters of gauze; 15,000 pounds (6,800 kg) of bandages; 30 gallons (113 L) of iodine; and 2,000 barrels of ether, along with leather gloves, Vaseline, cocoa, tobacco, and other "comforts for the treatment of the sick."[77] By the end of October, largely due to Schiff's fundraising, New York donors alone had raised $250,000.[78]

In Allied War Hospitals

On September 23, the Mercy Ship reached port in Falmouth, England, where two units debarked for a war hospital in Paignton.[79] The other nurses had time to visit the town, but were reluctant to accept invitations to people's homes given their neutral mission. None wanted to make a "false move" and be perceived as sympathetic or hostile to the British cause. "Silence, we decided, was golden, and we kept our thinking caps on straight and at the right angle when in the company of others, not only citizens of belligerent countries but of our own as well," wrote Volk.[80] The Russian units left the group and travelled to London, enjoying sightseeing and theater before heading to Kiev via Stockholm.[81] The ship then headed to Pauillac, France, where two units left for Pau, a town in the Pyrenees. The final stop was Rotterdam, where those serving in Germany and Austro–Hungary debarked.[82]

Once they arrived at their destinations, most Mercy Ship units encountered similar opportunities and challenges. First, most were feted by nobility and royalty. Second, they had to transform ill-suited buildings such as schools, casinos, private estates, and theaters into war hospitals. Third, they had to work with people who spoke different languages and adhered to different cultural norms. Fourth, most had leisure time to travel and sightsee, but sometimes felt frustrated with little to do. And last, many units were roiled by interpersonal conflicts.

The American Women's War Hospital in Paignton, where two units served, had already been established by a group of wealthy American expatriates at the vast country estate of American millionaire Paris Singer.[83] The eminent Sir William Osler, a founding professor at Johns Hopkins Hospital and now a professor of medicine at Oxford, served as the consulting surgeon for the hospital.[84] But these advantages were soon overshadowed by conflicts between physicians and nurses. The chief surgeon and director, Dr. Howard Beal of Worcester, Massachusetts, took an autocratic approach to hospital management. In a letter to the hospital's executive committee, Beal, a graduate of

Harvard Medical School who had served in the Spanish American war and Philippine occupation, stated that the chief surgeon's "will is absolute in all questions of medical care and procedure" including "the proper administration of such care and procedure."[85] This view clashed with that of the Matron (the British term for chief nurse), Australian nurse Gertrude Fletcher, who, following the norms of Anglo-American professional nursing, believed that she had charge of all nurses and nurse probationers in the hospital. It also undermined Delano's authority. ARC leaders had agreed that she would oversee all of the American nurses and she had instructed these nurses to write to her with their problems and concerns.[86] But Beal showed little respect for the nurses. In December 1914, he wrote Patterson asking whether the American nurses could be replaced with British ones, (whom he understood were paid much less). This way, the hospital would have enough funds to hire a pathologist—something Osler had recommended.[87] In January 1915, when the ARC sent all of the Mercy Ship nurses letters asking them if they wanted to renew their 6-month contract, some signed the contract but crossed out a portion saying that the ARC would not pay their return passage if they were discharged "for misconduct"—a likely indication of their frustration with the way they were being treated.[88] Meanwhile, the hospital had to send home the ARC's trained nurse anesthetist Grace Perkins, due to a British law stating that only a registered physician could perform anesthesia. Even Beal admitted to Patterson that Perkins had been "the most valuable nurse" in the hospital, and complained that the only replacement he could find was a retired doctor who had not performed anesthesia for 15 years but who demanded nearly double a nurse's salary.[89]

To make matters worse, the unit encountered 7 straight weeks of rain, followed by the winter freeze, and the members were quartered in poorly heated houses. Friction between Beal and the matron continued, and in April, she resigned, along with 12 American nurses and 3 British ones, and dared Beal to run the hospital without them.[90] In the interim, the Paignton unit faced "long periods of waiting" for casualties, who arrived periodically in trainloads an average of 10 days after leaving the front. However, the hospital reported only five deaths out of 1,905 cases—likely due to the triage systems the British were developing close to the front.[91] Despite this success and the excitement of a visit from Queen Mary in November 1914, work with the English unit made for a miserable experience that many sought to escape through periodic trips to London or transfers to other units.[92]

The two ARC medical units sent to Pau, in the South of France experienced better weather, more harmony, and finer accommodations, but initially faced a lack of work in buildings not initially suited to war medicine. Local leaders lent the ARC the Palais d'Hiver, a luxurious casino hotel that over-looked the white-capped Pyrenees, to use as a 200-bed war hospital.[93] The hotel featured a sunny palmarium at its center, which they converted into a dining room for convalescent patients.[94] The team soon moved in 166 long-term wounded soldiers who had been previously evacuated to the area, but received none directly from the far-away front. Despite the idyllic resort loca-tion, interest from a friendly Spanish marquesa who entertained nurses at her villa in Biarritz, weekend motor car jaunts to the mountains with local Amer-ican expatriates, and shopping trips to buy French lace, the nurses became restless from inactivity.[95]

It was not until late November, when wounded men began arriving in trainloads from the front, that the units began to feel useful. These men were "so dirty, so tired, so ragged, so sick, yet not one of them ready to admit that he is either hungry or exhausted or that his wound is more than a scratch," wrote head nurse Alice Henderson of Baltimore. Some patients arrived at the Pau hospital after 3 weeks in flooded trenches, with mud soaked uniforms and infected wounds embedded with bits of straw. Most were far from their families, so when a soldier died in the hospital, the units agreed that two nurses and one surgeon would attend each burial service.[96] But even with this routine of steady casualties and assigned mourning, many still felt far from the war. "It was almost like a city in a peaceful country," except for the soldiers and the women in black, wrote Baltimore nurse Vashti Bartlett in her unpublished memoir. "The gardens are full of flowers. The [bands are] playing in the park, there is food of every kind in plenty."[97] When the ARC called for nurses and doctors to replace medical personnel who had become infected during a typhus epidemic in Serbia, the whole Pau group volunteered. Patterson agreed to allow the hospital's director, Dr. Reynold M. Kirby-Smith of Sewanee, Tennessee, to go along with three nurses. In total, the Pau hospital treated only 598 patients, and its staff performed 225 major operations in its 11 months of existence.[98] When the hospital closed, Pau's Mayor thanked the ARC for developing "a very useful model for a great many of our sanitary formations," but ARC leaders believed the Pau units could have been more useful elsewhere.[99]

The two Kiev units, which crossed rough Baltic waters to reach their des-tination, encountered more work and greater obstacles to effectiveness. The Empress Dowager and other nobles greeted the units upon their arrival in Russia, and they later received a visit from the Tsar.[100] The surgeons were given Russian military uniforms and military officers' titles. The nurses were allowed to wear their Red Cross uniforms, but were also treated as an extension of the military and their letters were subject to government censorship. Oddly, the ARC did not object to this absorption of its personnel into a belligerent nation's military. Rather, Delano wrote in a January 1915 report, "This sounds all very business-like and assures us that the Russians have taken our units really as their very own."[101] Perhaps because their post lay remote from the watchful eyes of the Anglo-American press, and because the United States and Imperial Russia had cordial if distant relations, this unit seemed less concerned than others with maintaining the appearance of strict neutrality.

Of greater concern to the Kiev unit was the establishment of a modern, sanitary hospital. Once they arrived, the 25 ARC nurses, led by Hay, soon began scrubbing the floors and walls of the local Polytechnic institute, a cavernous building that the Russian government had lent to the ARC. "I think that Sister Helen eats scrub brushes," a Kiev hospital assistant reportedly told a *New York Tribune* correspondent.[102] While the building's high ceilings, many windows, and well-lit corridors made it a suitable modern hospital in most respects, all floors except the basement lacked running water after 10 a.m., and only the basement had hot water. The nurses addressed this problem by establishing a multi-stage system in which the entering patients, dirty and lice-ridden after weeks or months in the same uniform, were taken to the basement, stripped naked, had their hair shaved or cut, and beards clipped, then were bathed in hot water tubs before being transferred to a ward upstairs.[103] "When the new patients get here whether day or night, we all get up and give baths," Kiev nurse Aurel Baker wrote her family in Eagle, Wisconsin. "We have six bathtubs which can be used for the patients who are not badly hurt and we nurses take the sick ones to bathe."[104] The hospital employed a staff of "sanitars" —soldiers trained as hospital attendants—who performed the heavy work that hospital corpsmen and orderlies performed in US hospitals.[105] The sanitars bathed and groomed the ambulatory patients upon admission, freeing up the nurses to administer careful sponge baths for the seriously wounded.[106] Additionally, the unit created a "field disinfecting apparatus" for fumigating clothing, and established a thorough laundry system on the premises in which infected linens were soaked in antiseptic solutions before being cleaned, and in which sheets and linens were changed every 2–3 days.[107] The hospital's sanitary practices elicited interest from the Russians, and it soon began to receive as many visitors as patients.[108]

During the first months in Kiev, the physicians and nurses had regular schedules and leisure time. The nurses kept to 9-hour shifts, with two half days off per week.[109] Baker, who had worked as a supervisor at Chicago's Cook County Hospital after graduating from the Illinois Training School under Hay, wrote home, "[t]he work here reminds me of Cook County only it isn't nearly as hard. I have two very good men to help me so my work is to deal out medicine and watch. A Russian sister stays up to interpret."[110] The nurses and doctors took time to see the historic sites, explore the surrounding countryside, and meet locals. Nurse Eleanor Soukup, Baker's friend and Illinois Training School classmate, wrote to Baker's sister Alice, "the other day while watching a ball game, [Baker] became acquainted with a Russian; neither could speak the same language; she however, made an appointment with him with the aid of a calendar 1914." Soukup added "This makes the second time she almost became a citizen of this country on the hour a Cossack crossed her path; if I hadn't been with her she would have been captured."[111] Soukup herself stayed in Russia after the unit left, and married one of the unit's doctors, Dr. Brown McClintic of Peru, Indiana, in June 1916 while they were on duty with the Russian Army in Persia.[112] Dr. Philip Newton, another unit doctor, began a romance with a Russian volunteer nurse, Princess Helene Schahofskaya, and in January 1915, the two wed in Petrograd. The *New York Times* quoted Newton, a 1910 Graduate and Assistant professor of Anatomy at Georgetown Medical School, as saying that there was not enough work in the hospital so he "had nothing to do except fall in love."[113]

These relationships caused conflict within the unit. Most pointedly, Dr. Magill, who was married to a woman back in New York, openly flaunted his developing relationship with Camille Grandclement, a Russian princess and first Lieutenant in the Russian Medical Corps who was assisting in the hospital.[114] After Magill's disrespectful behavior on ship, this relationship provoked "outrage" among nurses, according to Farley.[115] Patterson subsequently telegraphed Magill to relieve him of his duties. Magill immediately joined the desperately short-staffed Russian Army Medical Corps as a Lieutenant General and headed to the front.[116] The following June, Magill would return to New York wearing his Russian uniform and his sword, and claim to have lost all but three of the 140 men under his command in a recent German advance. *The New York Times* article noting his flamboyant return also mentioned that his wife, Rose, had sued him for divorce the prior May "on statutory grounds" and that he had not contested the suit.[117] Given that the only statutory ground for divorce in New York was adultery, others in the unit (who received a clipping of this news in the mail) viewed the publication of Magill's highly public divorce and remarriage as damaging to their collective reputation. "Too bad it got out," Farley wrote in her diary.[118]

Even after Magill's removal, "bitter" differences continued to develop between Hay, the nurses, and the physicians. Ernest Bicknell, an ARC official who visited the hospital in spring 1915 with the Rockefeller Foundation's War Relief Commission, speculated that the "friction" stemmed from the clash between Hay's conservative standards for behavior and the more modern, looser ones of others in the unit.[119] (Presumably, she did not approve of the physicians' and nurses' flirtations and courtships.) Bicknell hoped that the arrival of Dr. Harry H. Snively, a Columbus, Ohio surgeon and National Guard Major who was slated to assume leadership of the hospital in April 1915, would smooth tensions.[120]

In spring 1915, the hospital staff suddenly had less time to focus on these social differences, due to an escalation in fighting between the Russians and Austro-Hungarians. In March, the Russians had captured a fortress at Przemyśl, and had taken 130,000 Austrians prisoner. This left the Russian Army free to attack the Austrians in the Carpathian mountains.[121] The Americans in Kiev shared in the celebration that accompanied these developments. Farley wrote in her diary March 22, "[w]e captured Peremishe [sic] today. Great rejoicing! That will about finish the Austrians." The next day she continued. "Everybody is hoping that the Peremishe [sic] victory will soon end the war." Though officially neutral, some American nurses, surrounded by rejoicing among their patients, began to identify with the Russians' cause.[122] But such identification took a somber turn when the casualties from the Russians' new campaign began streaming in to the Kiev hospital. "As soon as the Carpathian Campaign was in full swing, we were swamped with wounded," Dr. Arthur Zinkhan, a unit physician from Washington, D.C., later told American reporters.[123] On a single day in May, 13 trainloads of men arrived at the Kiev railroad station. All military hospitals were ordered to evacuate 8% of their patients every day and send them to the interior, regardless of their wounds.[124] The wards of the hospital filled up and patients spilled out into the corridors.[125] Snively performed as many as 15 operations a day.[126] The hospital expanded to 750 beds to absorb this overflow.[127] One of the hospital's elite Russian nurses, Marie Luise Von Koskull, wrote in her diary of the "great death"—a period of 10 days in May in which two to three soldiers died every night, and dead patients sometimes lay in their beds or on the floor for periods before the busy staff had time to remove them.[128] The unit's American doctors traveled to the front to try to persuade Russian military officials to allow them to move the hospital to Warsaw, close to the fighting, so they could treat the wounded more effectively. But the Russians politely rebuffed this idea.[129]

Just as the patient load was overwhelming the hospital's capacities, the staff dwindled. In early June, Hay resigned, likely due to the longstanding conflicts, and headed for Bulgaria to establish the long-promised hospital training school, while other nurses left for Serbia to assist in typhus relief or left for home.[130] In July, the ARC announced it was withdrawing all units from Europe by year's end, except those in Serbia and Belgium. Then in September, amid a feared invasion of the city by the Austro-Hungarian army, the Kiev hospital was forced to evacuate all patients and close its doors.[131]

The Kiev hospital admitted 4,050 patients during the nine and a half months it was open, and the staff performed nearly 1,000 major operations requiring anesthesia, along with approximately 53,000 minor surgical operations and dressings.[132] The most common injuries presented were thigh and leg wounds, followed by facial wounds, according to a 1916 article by Snively. Bullets caused more wounds than did shells—the opposite of the pattern later seen in the US Army on the Western Front, in which over two-thirds of wounds came from direct shell hits or shrapnel.[133] But the Kiev unit also encountered the same disfiguring facial wounds that became the grotesque signature of Great War combat. A sergeant "who had part his jaw and all of his tongue shot away" mounted a surprising recovery, and remained at the hospital afterwards to teach others with similar wounds how to eat and keep their faces clean, Minnegerode wrote ARC headquarters.[134]

Overall the Kiev hospital reported a mortality rate of 3.85%—much higher than that reported by other Mercy Ship hospitals.[135] This high mortality rate was likely caused by the conditions in which the patients arrived at the hospital, many days or even weeks after being wounded, "in a very depleted condition."[136] Although Russian doctors and nurses staffed trains that carried these soldiers from the front, they seldom changed dressings (likely due to lack of supplies) and anti-tetanus serum was unavailable. The Kiev hospital reported 3,497 Staphylococcus infections (over 86% of admissions!) and over 1,000 cases of osteomyelitis, a serious condition in which Staphylococcus bacteria has infected the bones.[137] This high rate of infection often prevented the physicians from operating. Dr. Dean Winn, an Atlanta doctor who joined the unit in December 1914, later reported that "most of the fractures of the arm and leg were literally bathed in pus by the time they reached us" and their "treatment was unsatisfactory and constructive treatment was impossible owing to the acute infection always present."[138] Neither could the doctors follow the patient for long periods due to the Russian Army's requirement to evacuate most patients to the interior to make room for new arrivals.[139]

This problem of infected wounds, caused by anaerobic bacteria from the rich agricultural soil of rural battlefields, was confronting medical teams in all belligerent nations. While surgeons traditionally favored a "conservative" approach of non-interference to allow infection to clear up on its own, some realized this approach was not working and began experimenting with more aggressive approaches to control infection. In late 1914, British military surgeon H.M.W. Gray had begun surgically excising infected wound tissue and a margin of non-infected tissue around it, while others were trying different antiseptic solutions either topically, or in the case of the Germans, intravenously. The debate over aggressive versus conservative treatment of infected combat wounds raged in medical journals throughout the first years of the war.[140] It is hardly surprising, then, that the overwhelmed American surgeons of the Kiev unit even experimented with applying gasoline to infected wounds.[141]

After the Kiev hospital closed, American expatriates in Petrograd raised funds for several nurses and doctors to remain. These expatriates believed that the nursing-medical units' departure from the Russian Empire at its time of greatest need was "humiliating and damaging to American interests"— especially businesses seeking to expand Russian operations and markets.[142] The expatriates' concerns turned to alarm when they later learned that 38 ARC nurses and nine doctors who had been working in German and Austro-Hungarian hospitals had come to Russia, under an arrangement between the German Red Cross and the ARC, to inspect the conditions of camps holding German and Austro-Hungarian prisoners.[143] Under a mutual agreement, the Russian government was supposed to send a similar team to German and Austro-Hungarian camps, but this part of the mission fell through. The presence of these Americans in Russia caring for enemy prisoners, at the same time as the Kiev unit withdrew, created "an impression that the American people were more solicitous about the health of the enemies of Russia than they were about the Russians themselves," a Petrograd expatriate wrote to leading Commerce Department officials. After the Commerce Department alerted the White House and ARC Headquarters to this possible diplomatic problem, ARC headquarters began supporting the Petrograd expatriates in their effort to keep some of the unit in Kiev.[144]

Three of the Mercy Ship physicians and five of the nurses remained for another year. For 2 months, they ran an evacuation hospital in Kiev, near the city's central train station. The hospital "received, dressed, cared for and evacuated either to the front or to interior hospitals" over 3,000 patients.[145] In November 1915, the Russian Army sent this group, along with eight Russian nursing sisters and nearly fifty *sanitars*, to work at a Russian Army hospital at Khoy in northern Persia.[146] The small group medically supported the Russian Army as it advanced toward Baghdad, then during its painful retreat. Its members returned to the United States in November 1916.[147]

In articles analyzing the Kiev operation, Snively and supervising nurse Lucy Minnegerode agreed that unit's work had offered them invaluable experience in establishing a war zone hospital.[148] They had organized a system for "handling large numbers of patients at once, all weary, ill, hungry and cold, and all anxious to get well as quickly as possible," Minnegerode noted.[149] This experience had also underlined the need for treatment of severely wounded combatants closer to the front. The British and American armies, responding to this need, were already developing more effective multi-tiered triage and treatment systems near the Western Front.[150] The Russians' answer to this problem became the flying column, a mobile tent hospital that moved with the Army. Several American Mercy Ship doctors went on to serve in these flying columns.[151]

Serving in Germany and Austria-Hungary

The experiences of the ARC units in Germany and Austria-Hungary in many respects resembled those of the units in Allied countries. The units were welcomed and celebrated by nobility; they converted ill-fitting public buildings into modern hospitals; and some doctors clashed with nurses, then were relieved or transferred for improper behavior such as misuse of Red Cross funds.[152] But unlike most units in the Allied nations, the Budapest, Kosel, Vienna, and Gleiwitz units had little leisure time once the hospitals opened: they treated wave after wave of horribly wounded men, and had to work up to 7 days a week.[153]

For the Budapest unit, the warm welcome accorded by the locals belied little difficulty and seemed to promise great adventure. The unit was initially quartered at the luxurious Astoria Hotel. Archduke Salvato, Austro-Hungarian Emperor Franz Joseph's son-in-law, paid a personal visit to the nurses as they worked to transform a boarding school for blind children into a war hospital.[154] But the veneer of luxury soon disappeared as the unit struggled to equip and operate a modern sanitary hospital in this charming but antiquated building. Not only were there no elevators, forcing the nurses and doctors to run up and down five flights of stairs, the building also lacked proper heating. They had to feel and guess at bone fractures until an X-ray machine was finally procured with the help of Countess Gladys Vanderbilt Széchenyi, the American expatriate heiress.[155] Moreover, they were met with an unrelenting stream of wounded men who, like their enemies the Russians, had been marinating in their infections during the long journey from the Eastern Front. "We puddled in pus," wrote Volk, who with her sister Rose was stationed in the Budapest hospital. "The wounds were reeking with stench, because they had had only first aid dressings applied, and had not been changed for days. There was no evidence of antiseptics having been used, and there was rotten sloughing skin, or gangrene, in nearly every use."[156]

An official report estimated the wound infection rate in Budapest to be 85% to 90%—similar to that in Kiev. However, the unit reported a low death rate of 1.5% (24 deaths out of 1,543 cases). Even more remarkable, the unit in Vienna, which operated a 400-bed hospital in a converted brick school-house, reported only 5 deaths in 2,050 cases (0.24% death rate). The low death rate in Vienna was likely because the patients' wounds, most commonly bullet wounds to the extremities (as in Kiev), were almost always only mildly infected, with no sepsis. This lack of infection was "due to the general use of iodine as a first aid dressing in the field," by the Austro-Hungarian army, according to a medical journal report by unit surgeon P.A. Smithe of Enid, Oklahoma.[157] The death rate, however, did not tell the whole story. Smithe's article includes pictures of grotesquely swollen limbs with mounds of protruding, scarred flesh, while nurses' writings describe shock at the sight of chest punctures that made visible the patient's breathing lung, or "a face with no eyes."[158] While these disfiguring wounds soon pervaded war hospitals in every belligerent nation, certain injuries seemed particular to Eastern and Southern Fronts. Volk described how the Budapest nurses unwrapped a patient in full uniform, whose feet had frozen solid and dropped off his legs during transportation. The patient died while the nurses were taking off his uniform.[159] Similarly, Sarah McCarron, a nurse in the unit stationed at Kosel, in Germany's northeast peninsula, wrote in her diary, "At 10 p.m. a transport case came in—seven men in Room 25, one man had his two feet frozen off. Both feet had been amputated (feet were frozen in Russia); was on the field 38 hours."[160] The nurses lamented that so many men with treatable injuries had been left to die in the snow, due to lack of treatment near the front and the shortage of resources to evacuate them.[161]

The nurses in Germany and Austria-Hungary also took greater care than those in Allied nations to assert their neutrality. According to Volk, Budapest residents could not distinguish between American and British accents, so it was very important for the nurses, when traveling in the city, to try to speak German or even the few words of Hungarian they knew. One group, speaking English on a tram car, was reprimanded for speaking an "enemy tongue."[162] On another occasion, Volk recalled being invited to tea at the home of Madam Jelen, a Hungarian socialite and singer, whose other guests included an Austro-Hungarian Prince. Madam Jelen showed Volk an autographed picture of the Kaiser, a prize possession that he had given her when she had sung for him. While being polite and appreciative, Volk had to make sure not to say the wrong thing. "This matter of representing America put us into a rather delicate position," she later wrote. "We could not be at ease: at all times we must be aware of the fact that we were heavily laden with the duties of an important mission—service. Neutral service!"[163]

Such care to stay neutral proved challenging. When Belgrade temporarily fell to the Central Powers in early December, the units in Germany and Austria were surrounded by victory celebrations. Bands were playing in the street all day and night, and patients were elated. "We Americans did not dare voice any sentiments in regard to the situation," Volk recalled.[164] McCarron's diary reflects this strenuous effort to remain detached. She recorded the fall of Belgrade and subsequent Central Powers victories in the same clinical, neutral tone she used to report her daily walks or patients' deaths. "They are celebrating another victory today," she wrote on December 17, 1914. "The Germans captured 16 Army Corps, that is, almost 1,000,000 men." The next day she corrected this figure to 300,000, but did not register any sentiment toward it. However, on Christmas night, McCarron noted with displeasure the way her unit director, Dr. Bial F. Bradbury of Norway, Maine, had diverted from strict neutrality during the dinner celebration at the hospital. "Was disgusted in the beginning to see our American flag draped below the German & under the Kaiser's picture & to cap the climax to hear Dr. Bradbury, our Chief, toast the Kaiser first & President Wilson second. The dinner was a long drawn-out affair for me."[165]

It is not surprising that the obedience-trained nurses showed more concern for adhering to the rules of neutrality than did the doctors. However, even McCarron and Volk, whose writings indicate strenuous efforts to remain neutral, showed signs of slipping in places. McCarron celebrated the Kaiser's birthday, a national holiday, and sent war postcards of the Kaiser and his family home to her nieces and nephews in Brooklyn. On a February 1915 postcard of the four Kronprinzes addressed to her nephew, she wrote "Aren't these boys nice?"[166] Similarly, Volk apparently saw no problem with developing friendly relationships with her Austro-Hungarian patients and accepting parts of their uniforms as mementos. On one occasion, she incurred the wrath of her supervisor, Alice Beattie, who wrote Delano to report walking into Volk's room and finding Volk in a Kimono with a patient who had just been discharged, wearing his soldier's cap. Volk's sister Rose, also a Mercy Ship nurse, was in the room with them (and according to Volk's own account, Volk was sick in bed). When Beattie "reproved" them, both Volks refused to acknowledge that their behavior had been improper. According to Volk, this had been a special visit by a grateful patient to present the cap. But Volk and her sister's refusal to be embarrassed only fueled Beattie's conviction that Volk was "totally misfitted" for war nursing and had "no conception of the dignity of her profession or the dignity of a woman."[167] Volk was nevertheless allowed to remain for the remainder of her 6-month term, and left only because she was diagnosed with rheumatoid arthritis in her hands and feet as well as a heart murmur, likely worsened by the long days running up and down the five flights of stairs in the Budapest hospital.[168]

A final difficulty with neutrality surfaced just before the ARC units left Germany and Austria-Hungary. Soon after the Budapest nurses and surgeons learned that they were to be awarded medals in a ceremony presided over by the Archduke, Boardman sent them a letter from ARC headquarters stating that they were forbidden as neutrals from accepting any decorations from a foreign government. She eventually changed her mind, and allowed the unit to accept their medals.[169] Boardman nevertheless raised no objections when the Russian government in 1915 awarded all of the Kiev nurses St. Anne's Cross, the highest award for civilian service.[170] This inconsistency might have reflected a realization that American public opinion was turning away from the Central Powers. It did not, however, reflect an explicit choice at ARC head-quarters to move away from neutrality. The organization's publications in 1915 and 1916, which were distributed to a growing membership in the United States, devoted just as much space to articles describing Red Cross work in the Central Powers as they did to Red Cross work on the Allied side.[171] Despite the effective Allied blockade, the ARC supported the efforts of prominent German- and Austrian-Americans to supply war hospitals in these countries, right up to the severing of relations between these countries and the United States in early 1917.[172]

Returning Home

Most of the original Mercy Ship nurses and physicians remained in the war zone for a year or more. While the ARC sent groups of replacement personnel over in March 1915, a greater proportion of the physicians than nurses had to be replaced. Overall, the nurses stayed an average of nearly 46 days more than the physicians.[173] Among those nurses who remained through October 1915, when the ARC recalled all units, some then transferred to the American Ambu-lance, a Paris war hospital supported by the American expatriate community, or remained to work with other nations' Red Cross societies or militaries.[174] A few did not leave the war zone until 1919, and many returned to it in 1917 to serve with the US forces in France.[175] Reba Taylor, a nurse in the Paignton, England unit, fell ill and died soon after she returned home to Washington, D.C. In an official ARC publication, Taylor's death was attributed to her "thir-teen months of arduous service, day and night."[176] While this may have been an exaggeration, given that the Paignton unit experienced slack periods, some nurses were worn down by the psychological strain of witnessing unrelenting suffering. "We don't say much about it," Louise Bennett, a supervising nurse at Paignton, wrote nurses at ARC headquarters, "but we are all heartily sick of this endless cruelty and wickedness."[177] Volk added in her memoir: "Some persons think that doctors and nurses get used to the presence or imminence of death, with its attendant suffering and sorrow. But such is not the case." Instead, she noted that doctors and nurses learn to suppress their emotions, which at times causes "a severe strain, both physically and mentally." While service at war hospitals had turned a few participants into partisans for the nations where they served, it had turned many against the war altogether.

Back home, Americans had seemingly lost patience with Europe's war. The ARC had raised over $1.2 million for the Mercy Ship and related units, but fundraising lagged by mid-1915, leading the ARC to decide call the units home by October.[178] The May 7, 1915 sinking of the *R.M.S. Lusitania*, in which 128 Americans died, had swung American sympathies toward the Allies, making war relief that involved aid to Germany much less popular with many.[179] The German blockade of Allied ships, which had begun in February 1915, had also made it difficult for the ARC to continue to send medical supplies and other relief items to hospitals in the Central Powers, although it continued to try to negotiate a way to do so through mid-1916.[180] In 1917, when the United States entered the First World War on the side of the Allies, the ARC finally abandoned neutrality in favor of patriotism and became a supportive auxiliary of the American Expeditionary Forces.[181]

Conclusion

The ARC's Mercy Ship served as an important demonstration of the United States' good faith effort at neutral humanitarian engagement in the First World War, during a time when the meaning of neutrality in warfare appeared fluid, and the rules for staying neutral did not seem clear. The ARC nurses and doctors became able ambassadors for modern hospital organization, surgical techniques, and for instituting what Dr. Smithe of the Vienna unit called "an antiseptic conscience" in operating rooms and wound dressing areas.[182] In Kiev, Russia and southern France, areas that had little prior exposure to these methods, the ARC units introduced a modern model of war medicine. More generally, the mission demonstrated that the ARC could use nursing and medical assistance as a form of effective humanitarian engagement. Moreover, while humanitarian organizations had previously sent doctors to battlefields, the preeminence of nurses in the Mercy Ship set a new precedent for war relief. As Delano stated at the ARC Annual Meeting in December 1915, "we have learned that women can be mobilized without confusion, that their chances of illness when carefully selected seem to be no greater than men's and that they face danger with equanimity." She also noted that the experiences in Europe had provided the nursing leaders with information about which kind of nurse is "most desirable" for war service.[183] When the United States entered the war on the side of the Allies in April 1917, the ARC nursing committee, unlike the US military, was already prepared to send its personnel "Over There."[184]

Notes

1. Lavinia L. Dock, Sarah Elizabeth Pickett, Clara D. Noyes, Fannie F. Clement, Elizabeth G. Fox, and Anna R. Van Meter, *History of American Red Cross Nursing* (New York: MacMillan, 1922), 139.

2. Jane E. Delano, "The Nurses and the Requirements;" 9): 225–29; "American Surgeons are Picked for the Field," *American Red Cross Magazine* 9, no. 4 (October 1914): 230–31.

3. Robert U. Patterson, "Annual Report of the Bureau of Medical Services for the Year 1915," in American National Red Cross, *Eleventh Annual Report of the American Red Cross, 1915* (Washington: American National Red Cross, 1916), 19–27.

4. The Conventions did not address civilians until the 1949 revisions. John F. Hutchinson, *Champions of Charity: War and the Rise of the Red Cross* (Boulder, CO: Westview Press, 1996), 46–50.

5. Kendrick A. Clements, "Woodrow Wilson and World War I," *Presidential Studies Quarterly* 34, no. 1 (March 2004): 66–70.

6. Lynn Dumenil, *The Second Line of Defense: American Women and World War I* (Chapel Hill, NC: University of North Carolina Press, 2017), 13.

7. United States Department of Veterans Affairs"America's Women Veterans: Military Service History and VA Benefit Utilization Statistics," (Washington, D.C: Department of Veterans Affairs, 2012, 2018), 2. accessed June 21, 2018, https://www.va.gov/vetdata/docs/SpecialReports/Final_Womens_Report_3_2_12_v_7.pdf.

8. Marian Moser Jones, *The American Red Cross from Clara Barton to the New Deal* (Baltimore, MD: Johns Hopkins University Press, 2013), 165; Dumenil, *The Second Line of Defense*, 1–2.

9. Dumenil, *The Second Line of Defense*, 14.

10. See, for example, Jeffrey S. Reznick, *Healing the Nation: Soldiers and the Culture of Caregiving during the Great War* (New York: Manchester University Press, 2004); Mark Harrison, *The Medical War: British Military Medicine in the First World War* (New York: Oxford University Press, 2010); Ana Carden-Coyne, *The Politics of Wounds: Military Patients and Medical Power in the First World War* (New York: Oxford, 2014); Emily Mayhew, *Wounded: A New History of the Western Front in World War I* (New York: Oxford, 2014); Sophie Delaporte, *Les Médecins dans la Grande Guerre: 1914–1918* (Paris: Bayard, 2003).

11. See, for example, Christine E.Hallett, *Containing Trauma: Nursing Work in the First World War* (Manchester, UK: Manchester Univeristy Press, 2011); Hallett, *Veiled Warriors: Allied Nurses of the First World War* (New York: Oxford University Press, 2014); Hallett

and Allison Fell, *First World War Nursing: New Perspectives* (New York: Routledge, 2013); Laurie S. Stoff, *Russia's Sisters of Mercy and the Great War: More than Binding Men's Wounds* (Lawrence, KS: University of Kansas Press, 2015).

12. Patricia D'Antonio, *American Nursing: A History of Knowledge, Authority and the Meaning of Work* (Baltimore: Johns Hopkins University Press, 2010), 28–79; Susan Reverby, *Ordered to Care: The Dilemma of American Nursing, 1850–1945* (New York: Cambridge University Press, 1987), 60.

13. George W. Crile and William E. Lower, *Surgical Shock and the Shockless Operation through Anoci-Association* (Philadelphia, PA: W.B. Saunders, 1914).

14. Marianne Bankert, *Watchful Care: A History of America's Nurse Anesthetists* (New York: Continuum, 1989), 40–44; D'Antonio, *American Nursing*, 62–63.

15. Nancy F. Cott, *Public Vows: A History of Marriage and the Nation* (Cambridge, MA: Harvard University Press, 2000), 159–60.

16. Jones, *The American Red Cross*, 34, 38.

17. Ibid., 80–81.

18. Ibid., 112–13.

19. Charles Lynch, "Report of Maj. Charles Lynch, Medical Department, General Staff, U.S. Army, Observer with the Japanese Forces in Manchuria," in *Reports of Military Observers Attached to the Armies in Manchuria during the Russo-Japanese War, Part 4* (Washington: GPO, 1907), 58–61.

20. Jones, *The American Red Cross*, 167.

21. Dock et al., *History of ARC Nursing*, 78–79.

22. D'Antonio, *American Nursing*, 29–30.

23. Dock et al., *History of ARC Nursing*, 78–79.

24. Delano to Mabel T. Boardman, September 12, 1912, Folder 140.1 Nursing Service Bureau of Instructions, Box 18, Group 1, Records of the American National Red Cross, Record Group 200, National Archives and Records Administration, College Park, MD. (Hereafter RG 200, NACP).

25. Reverby, *Ordered to Care*, 36.

26. Ibid., 53.

27. Darlene Clark Hine, *Black Women in White: Racial Conflict and Cooperation in the Nursing Profession, 1890–1950* (Bloomington: Indiana University Press, 1989), 26–27, 47.

28. Dock et al., *History of American Red Cross Nursing*, 405–6.

29. Jones, *The American Red Cross*, 142–43.

30. "Robert Urie Patterson," Arlington National Cemetery website website, http://www.arlingtoncemetery.net/rupatterson.htm. Accessed June 3, 2019,

31. Robert U. Patterson, "The American National Red Cross in First Aid and Accident Prevention," *Maryland Medical Journal* 59, no. 6 (June 1916): 133.

32. Mabel T. Boardman, "The Story of the Ship;" Boardman, "The Appeals for Europe's Wounded," both in *ARC Magazine* 9, no. 4 (October 1914): 209–17.

33. Delano, Fifth Annual Report of the National Committee on Red Cross Nursing, December 1914. Folder 140.1 Nursing Service, Box 18, Grp 1, RG 200, NACP.

34. Fay Shriver, "Helen Scott Hay/Clara D. Noyes: Department of Red Cross Nursing," *American Journal of Nursing (hereafter AJN)* 33, no. 1 (January 1933): 67–69.

35. Delano, "The Nurses and the Requirements," 225–29; Dock et al., *History of ARC Nursing*, 142.

36. Memo, ARC Division of Information, 1915, Folder, 591.4 ARC Medical Units Personnel, Box 18, Grp 1, RG 200 NACP. U.S. House, *Tenth Annual Report of the American National Red Cross*, 63d Cong. 2d sess., 1915, H. Doc. 1665, 21.

37. Jane A. Delano, "The Red Cross," *AJN* 15, no. 1 (October 1914): 36; "Passport Applications," National Archives and Research Administration website, accessed June 25, 2018, http://www.archives.gov/research/passport/.

38. Chad E. O'Lynn, "History of Men in Nursing: A Review," in *Men in Nursing: History, Challenges, and Opportunities*, ed. O'Lynn and Russell E. Tranbarger (New York: Springer, 2007), 25–27.

39. Boardman to Mrs. Whitelaw Reid, August 12, 1914, Folder 591.4 Medical Relief Units –France, Box 18, Grp 1, RG 200, NACP.

40. Delano, "The Red Cross," *AJN* 15, no. 2 (1914): 127.

41. Dock et al., *History of ARC Nursing*, 142.

42. Katherine Volk, *Buddies in Budapest* (Los Angeles: Kellaway-Ide Co, 1936), 31.

43. Lucy Minnegerode Diary, 1914–15, 131, ARC Archives, Washington, DC; Dock et al., *History of ARC Nursing*, 142.

44. *Tenth Annual Report of the ARC*, 20. Memo, ARC Division of Information, 1915, Folder, 591.4 ARC Medical Units Personnel, Box 18, Grp 1, RG 200, NACP.

45. Paul Starr, *The Social Transformation of American Medicine: The Rise of a Sovereign Profession and the Making of a Vast Industry* (New York: Basic Books, 1982), 123–25.

46. Boardman to Herman Harjes, July 28, 1915, Folder 591.4 Medical Units- General, Box 18, Grp 1, RG 200 NACP.

47. Ibid.

48. Patterson, "Information for Directors of Units Regarding the Official Relations of the Surgeons and Nurses with American Red Cross in Europe," February 24, 1915, Folder 591.4 Medical Units- General, Box 18, Grp 1, RG 200, NACP.

49. Dock et al., *History of ARC Nursing*, 143–44; Delano, "The Nurses and the Requirements," 226; Delano, "The Red Cross," *AJN* 15, no. 1 (October 1914): 37.

50. "Chronology," Folder 4, Series 2, Sarah McCarron papers, Barbara Bates Center for the Study of the History of Nursing, University of Pennsylvania School of Nursing.

51. Dock et al., *History of Red Cross Nursing*, 142; Delano, "The Nurses and the Requirements," 226.

52. Minnegerode Diary, September 3, 1914, ARC.

53. Ross J. Wilson, *New York and the First World War: Shaping an American City* (New York: Routledge, 2016), 91–92.

54. Judith S. Graham, ed., *"Out Here at the Front": The World War One Letters of Nora Saltonstall* (Boston: Northeastern University Press, 2004), 7; Dumenil, *The Second Line of Defense*, 106.

55. Dock et al., *History of ARC nursing*, 144; Boardman, "The Story of the Ship," 213; Minnegerode Diary, 34–68, ARC. Mary Frederika Farley, Diary, Sept. 17–18, 1914; Folder 1, Mary Frederika Farley papers, Radcliffe Schlesinger Library, Harvard University.

56. Sarah McCarron diary, September 10–11, 1914, McCarron Papers, Bates Center.

57. The Red Cross did not exclude Jewish nurses from service. A list of those who served in a German unit notes that two are "R. Catholic." The remaining are listed as

"Protestant." See "American Red Cross Assigned to Service in Germany," Folder 591.4, Nurses Medical Relief Unit–Germany, Box 18, Grp 1, RG 200, NACP.

58. Minnegerode Diary, September, 1914, undated, 12–14, ARC.

59. Ibid., September 7, 1914.

60. Charlotte Perry, "Nursing Ethics and Etiquette," *AJN* 6, no. 7 (June 1906): 451–52.

61. Vashti Bartlett, "Duties of Junior Nurse," c. 1903–1906, Folder "Student Notebook Johns Hopkins Hospital Practical Nursing, GYN, Materia Medica, Miss Freese," Box 2, Bartlett Papers, Collections of the William H. Welch Medical Library, Johns Hopkins University (JHU).

62. Reverby, *Ordered to Care*, 54–56.

63. Starr, "The Social Transformation of American Medicine," 141–44.

64. Farley Diary, September 18–19, 1914, Schlesinger.

65. Ibid., September 16, 1914.

66. Ibid.

67. Dr. Robert U. Patterson to Dr. Howard Beal, 29 December, 1914, Folder 591.4. Medical Relief Units Paignton, England Box 18, Grp 1, RG 200, NACP.

68. Volk, *Buddies in Budapest*, 32, 36, 39, 113–14, 138.

69. Ibid., 136.

70. Boardman, "The Story of the Ship," 209; Dock et al., *History of ARC Nursing*, 143.

71. "Red Cross Held for Neutral Crew : Captain's Proposal to Hold Germans on Board Rejected by U.S.," *New York Tribune*, September 10, 1914, 7; "Mercy Ship Gets American Crew: Sailing of Red Cross To-day Still Awaits Federal Consent," *New York Tribune*, September 11, 1914, 7; Boardman, "The story of the ship," 212.

72. Boardman, "Story of the Ship," 210–11; "Germans on Crew Delay Start of Red Cross," *San Francisco Chronicle*, September 13, 1914, 31.

73. Volk, *Buddies in Budapest*, 48–49.

74. Boardman, "Story of the Ship"; "Red Cross Waits to Parade River: Mercy Ship Delays Sailing a Day so New Yorkers Can See Her," *New York Tribune*, September 7, 1914, 7.

75. Minnegerode Diary, September 7, 1914, ARC.

76. Sherman Montrose Craiger, "Our Christmas Ships," *The Sun*, December 20, 1914, SM3.

77. Dock et al., *History of ARC Nursing*, 141.

78. "Red Cross Held for Neutral Crew," 7; Wilson, *New York and the First World War*, 91.

79. Delano, "The Red Cross," *AJN* 15, no. 3 (December 1914): 205.

80. Volk, *Buddies in Budapest*, 46–47.

81. Farley Diary, October 1–5, 1914, Schlesinger.

82. Dock et al., *History of ARC Nursing*, 145, 150; Craiger, "Our Christmas Ships," SM3.

83. Louise S. Heyen, "From the War Zone," *Trained Nurse and Hospital Review* 24, no. 5 (November 1915): 287.

84. U.S. House, *Eleventh Annual Report of the American National Red Cross for the Year 1915*, 64th Cong., 1st sess., 1915, H. Doc. 1307, 13; "Report of the Central committee

January 1, 1916," 11; Folder Excerpts from Central and Executive Committee Minutes, 1905–1916, Box 18, Grp 1, RG 200, NACP.

85.   Dr. Howard Beal to the Executive Committee, American Women's War Relief Fund, Undated, Folder 591.4 Medical Relief Units–Paignton, England. Box 18, Grp 1, RG 200, NACP; M. A. DeWolfe Howe, "Howard Walter Beal," in *Memoirs of the Harvard Dead in the War against Germany*, vol. 3 (Cambridge, MA: Harvard University Press, 1922), 504–05.

86.   Boardman to Mrs. Harcourt, June 1, 1915; Howard Beal, "American Red Cross Report for April 1915," both in Folder 591.4 Medical Relief Units–Paignton, England. Box 18, Grp 1, RG 200, NACP; Dock et al., *History of ARC Nursing*, 147.

87.   Beal to Patterson, December 10,1914, Folder 591.4 Medical Relief Units–Paignton, England, Box 18, Grp 1, RG 200, NACP.

88.   Beal to Patterson, January 28, 1915; Louise A. Bennett, signed contract; Folder 591.4 Medical Relief Units–Paignton, England, Box 18, Grp 1, RG 200, NACP.

89.   Beal, American Red Cross Report for January 1915; Beal to Patterson, January 4, 1915, Folder 591.4 Medical Relief Units–Paignton, England, Box 18, Grp 1, RG 200, NACP.

90.   Beal, ARC Report for April 1915, Folder 591.4, Box 18, Grp 1, RG 200, NACP.

91.   "Statistical Report from Opening of Hospital to 1st October, 1915," Folder 591.4 Medical Relief Units Paignton, England. Box 18, Grp 1, RG 200, NACP; *Eleventh Annual Report of ARC* 16; Harrison, *The Medical War*, 26.

92.   Dock et al., *History of ARC Nursing*, 146–49; "Word from the Front," *ARC Magazine* 10, no. 1 (January 1915): 37.

93.   Vashti Bartlett, "Pau," Folder "Diary march 25 1915–January 1916," Box 7, Bartlett Papers, JHU.

94.   Jane A. Delano, "A Chat about the Nurses Abroad," *ARC Magazine* 10, no. 2 (February 1915): 81–83.

95.   Bartlett Diary, May 23, 1915; V. Bartlett to Alice Bartlett, letters, June 1915 to August 1915, Folder Correspondence to sister Alice Bartlett, JHU.

96.   Henderson to Delano, November 1914, in Dock et al., *History of ARC Nursing*, 151. Bartlett to "Mother," June 2, 1915. JHU.

97.   Bartlett, "Pau," Folder Diary March 25, 1915–January 1916, Box 7, JHU.

98.   *ARC Annual Report 1915*, 9–10.

99.   "Word from the Front," 41. Acting Chairman, (Boardman), to Mr. Thomas Newbold, September 2, 1915. Folder 591.4 Medical Relief Units General, Box 18, Grp 1, RG 200, NACP.

100.   "Honor Paid to U.S. Red Cross Corps on the Way to Duty at Kief, Russia," *Washington Post*, October 12, 1914, 2; Lucy Minnegerode, "The Red Cross: Experiences of Unit C at Kief, Russia," *AJN* 16, no. 3 (December 1915): 220–24.

101.   Delano, "The Red Cross," *AJN* 15, no. 4 (January 1915): 302.

102.   Alice O. Beattie to Delano, March 1, 1915, Folder 591.4 Medical Relief Units Austria & Hungary, Box 18, Grp 1. RG 200, NACP.

103.   Minnegerode, "The Red Cross," 222–23.

104.   Aurel Baker to "My Dear Mother," April 16/29, 1915, Folder "Letters Through 1915," Aurel Baker Pardee Papers, Wisconsin Historical Society, Madison, Wisc.

105.   "Army Hospital Corps : A Member of the Hospital Corps with the Russian Army," *Meyer Brothers Druggist* 27, no. 1 (January 1906): 12.

106. Minnegerode, "The Red Cross," 223.

107. Maj. H. H. Snively, "Base Hospital Work in Russia," *Military Medicine* 38, no. 6 (June 1916): 627.

108. Minnegerode, "The Red Cross," 222.

109. Ibid., 224.

110. Aurel Baker to "My Dear Mother", April 16/29, 1915, Baker Pardee Papers, Wisconsin.

111. Eleanor Soukup to Alice Baker, Baker Pardee Papers, Wisconsin.

112. "Nursing News and Announcements," *AJN* 19, no. 4 (January 1919): 323.

113. "Red Cross Surgeon Weds," *New York Times*, January 23, 1915, 3; "American Red Cross Doctors and Nurses in Russia," *Christian Advocate* 82 (October 1915): 14; Joshua Segal, "American Humanitarian Volunteerism in Russia's Military 1914–1917," (Doctoral diss., George Washington University, 2018), 14.

114. "American Surgeons Are Picked for the Field," 230; Camille G. Magill, "Obituary," *News Journal*, September 3, 1928, 3.

115. Farley Diary, October 17, 1914, Schlesinger.

116. "Dr. Magill Back from War," *New York Times*, June 16, 1915, 14; Sagal, "American Humanitarian Volunteerism," 15; Stoff, *Russia's Sisters of Mecy*, 44.

117. "Dr. Magill Back from War."

118. Farley Diary, April 2, 1915, Schlesinger; Cott, *Public Vows*, 195.

119. Segal, "American Humanitarian Volunteerism," Ch. 1, 45; citing Bicknell to Boardman, June 7, 1915, Folder 900.2, RG 200, NACP.

120. Ibid.; Snively, "Base Hospital Work in Russia," 623.

121. Segal, "American Humanitarian Volunteerism," Ch. 1, 40; citing David R. Stone, *The Russian Army in the Great War: The Eastern Front, 1914–1917* (Lawrence, MA: University of Kansas Press, 2015), 144.

122. Farley Diary, March 22–23, 1915, Schlesinger.

123. Segal, "American Humanitarian Volunteerism," Ch. 1, 45; citing "American Nurses Return from War Zone; Worked Under Guns," *Oakland Tribune*, November 9, 1915, 6.

124. Segal, "American Humanitarian Volunteerism," Ch. 1, 46; citing Harry Hamilton Snively and J. George Frederick, eds., *The Battle of the Non-Combatants; the letters of Dr. Harry Hamilton Snively to his family from Russia, Poland, France, Belgium, Persia, etc., Assembled by His Daughter, Marjorie Knowlton Snively* (New York: The Business bourse, 1933), 22, 29.

125. Aurel Baker to "Folks at Home," May 10, 1915, Baker Pardee Papers, Wisconsin Library.

126. Segal, "American Humanitarian Volunteerism," Ch. 1, 48; citing Snively, *Battle of the Non-Combatants*, 27.

127. Snively, "Base Hospital work in Russia," 623.

128. Ibid., 50; citing Marie Luise Baronin Von Koskull, *Damals in Russland* (Leipzing, Germany: Berleght bei Koehler & Umelang, 1931), 50; Von Kuskull was a Baltic German noblewoman, whose family was loyal to the Russian Empire.

129. Segal, "American Humanitarian Volunteerism," Ch. 1, 42–43; citing Dr. Edward Egbert to U.S. Ambassador, Petrograd, March 24, 1915; Ministry of Foreign Affairs to U.S. Ambassador, Petrograd, March 24, 1915, Folder 814.2 U.S. Embassy

Russia, Record Groups of the Foreign Service Posts of the Department of State, RG 84, NACP.

130. Dock et al., *History of ARC Nursing*; Rachel C. Torrance to Snively, May 26, 1915. Folder 591.4 Medical Relief Units Russia, Box 18, Grp 1, RG 200, NACP. 158.

131. Snively, "Base Hospital Work in Russia," 632.

132. Ibid.; *ARC Annual Report 1915*, 17.

133. "Battle Casualties, 1917 and 1918 in the American Expeditionary Forces: Table 22. Wounds by Gunshot missiles, World War," in *Report of the Surgeon General U.S. Army to the Secretary of War* (Washington: G.P.O, 1920), 63.

134. Dock et al., *History of ARC Nursing*, 158.

135. Snively, "Base Hospital Work in Russia," 633; *ARC Annual Report 1915*, 14, 16; "Statistical Report from Opening of Hospital to 1st October, 1915," Folder 591.4 Medical Relief Units Paignton, England, Box 18, Grp 1, RG 200, NACP.

136. *ARC Annual Report 1915*, 18.

137. Snively, "Base Hospital Work in Russia," 625, 637.

138. Dean F. Winn, ""Statistical Report of Five Hundred and Seventy Cases Treated in the American Red Cross Hospital at Kiev Russia," *Military Surgeon* 38, no. 1 (January 1916): 63.

139. Ibid.

140. Harrison, *The Medical War*, 27–30.

141. Snively, "Base Hospital Work in Russia," 630.

142. Memo, unsigned, to Secretary of Commerce William Cox Redfield, quoting Petrograd Commercial Attaché Henry D. Baker, Sep 23, 1915, Folder 591.4 Medical Relief Units Russia, Box 18, Grp 1, RG 200, NACP; Segal, "American Humanitarian Volunteerism," Ch. 1, 68–69.

143. Donna G. Burgar and Katrina E. Hertzer, "Letters from Red Cross Nurses," *AJN* 16, no. 2 (November, 1915): 134–36; Henry D. Baker, to Chief, Bureau of Foreign and Domestic Commerce, U.S. Department of Commerce, November 8, 1915. Folder 591.4 Medical Relief Units Russia, Box 18, Grp 1, RG 200, NACP.

144. Memo to Secretary of Commerce, September 23, 1915; President Woodrow Wilson to Boardman, September 20, September 22, 1915; Boardman to J.P. Tumulty, Sept. 23, 1915; Baker to Chief, Bureau of Foreign and Domestic Commerce; Folder 591.4 Medical Relief Units Russia, Box 18, Grp 1, RG 200, NACP.

145. Snively, "Base Hospital Work in Russia," 632.

146. Dock et al., *History of ARC Nursing*, 159.

147. Segal, "American Humanitarian Volunteerism," Ch. 2, 2; Sean McMeekin, *Russian Origins of the First World War* (Cambridge, MA: Belknap Press of Harvard University, 2011), 189. citing McMeekin.

148. Snively, "Base Hospital Work in Russia," 623.

149. Minnegerode, "The Red Cross," 226.

150. Harrison, *The Medical War*, 32–41.

151. Segal, "American Humanitarian Volunteerism," Ch. 1, 84.

152. Patterson to Beal, Dec. 29, 1914; *ARC Annual Report 1915*, 16; Alice C. Beattie to Delano, March 3, 1915. Folder 591.4 Medical Relief Units Austria-Hungary, Box 18, Grp 1, RG 200 NACP.

153. McCarron diary, October 22–25, 1914; Volk, *Buddies in Budapest*, 130.

154. Volk, *Buddies in Budapest*, 99–100.

155. Ibid., 139.

156. Ibid., 112.

157. *ARC Annual Report 1915*, 14–16; P. A. Smithe, "With the American Red Cross in Vienna," *New York Medical Journal* 103, no. 7 (February 12, 1916): 301-305.

158. Ibid., 6–8; Volk, *Buddies in Budapest*, 141–42, 112–13, 137.

159. Volk, *Buddies in Budapest*, 136.

160. McCarron Diary, December 28, 1914.

161. Volk, *Buddies in Budapest*, 215.

162. Ibid., 97.

163. Ibid., 218.

164. Ibid., 157.

165. McCarron Diary, December 17, 18, 25, 1914; "American Surgeons Are Picked for the Field," 231.

166. Ibid., January 27, 1915; Postcard, Sarah McCarron to G. Henninger, February 26, 1915. Miscellaneous Postcards, McCarron Papers, Bates Center.

167. Alice Beattie to Delano, March 1, 1915, Folder 591.4 Medical Relief Units Austria-Hungary, Box 18, Grp 1, RG 200 NACP; Volk, *Buddies in Budapest*, 202.

168. Beattie to Delano, March 1, 1915; Volk, *Buddies in Budapest*, 203.

169. Ibid.; Volk, *Buddies in Budapest*, 227.

170. "American Nurses Decorated for Valor," *Red Cross Bulletin* 3, no. 2 (January 6, 1919), 8; Segal, "American Humanitarian Volunteerism," Ch. 1, 87.

171. For ARC's continued work in the Central Powers, see "A Letter from Munich," *ARC Magazine* 10, no. 1 (January 1915): 29; "German and Austro-Hungarian Relief in Chicago," *ARC Magazine* 11, no. 1 (January 1916): 47–49; "A Hospital that Holds On," *ARC Magazine* (November 1916): 369–74 (ARC Hospital in Munich).

172. Col. Jefferson R. Kean, ARC, to Dr. Frederic Kammerer, November 10, 1916; Kean to Julius Goldzier, November 23, December 4, 15, 1916, Telegram January 31, 1917; Goldzier to Kean, November 26, 1916, Telegrams December 1, 1916, January 31, 1917, February 7, 1917; Folder 591.4 Medical Relief Units Austria & Hungary, Box 18, Grp 1, RG 200, NACP.

173. "Period of Service for Nurses in Europe"; List of Physicians with dates of service, Folder 591.4 Medical Relief Units–General, Box 18, Grp 1, RG 200, NACP. This calculation excludes the few personnel who remained after all ARC units withdrew. Including this group, the nurses stayed on average 48.7 more days than the doctors.

174. Bartlett to Alice Bartlett, August 18, 1915, Bartlett Papers, JHU; Snively, "Base Hospital Work in Russia,"632; P. A. Smithe, "With the American Red Cross in Vienna," *New York Medical Journal* (February 12, 1916), Reprint, in 591.4 Medical Relief Units Austria & Hungary, Box 18, Grp 1, RG 200, NACP.

175. Aurel Baker Pardee, Register, p. 2, Pardee Papers, Wisc. Historical Society; "Florence May Cooper, *Reading Times*, April 7, 1919, 8; "Florence Cooper Dies; Retired Nurse was 93," *Baltimore Sun*, May 13, 1982, E4; Sarah McCarron, U.S. Army Nurse Corps service Record, Series 2, Folder 6, McCarron Papers, Bates Center.

176. "Another Life for Humanity," *ARC Magazine* 11, no. 2 (February 1916): 59.

177. Dock et al., *History of ARC Nursing*, 149.

178. Woodrow Wilson and William Howard Taft, "An Appeal," November 24, 1915, reprinted in *ARC Magazine* 11, no. 1 (January 1916): 17; Delano, "The Red Cross," 1111.

179. Michael S. Nieberg, *The Path to War: How the First World War Created Modern America* (New York: Oxford University Press, 2016), 67–71.

180. "Solution of Blockade Problem is Hoped for," *ARC Magazine* 11, no. 9 (September 1916): 329.

181. Jones, *The American Red Cross*, 159.

182. Smithe, "With the American Red Cross in Vienna," 305.

183. Delano, "A Stellar Red Cross Meeting," *ARC Magazine* 11, no. 1 (January 1916): 18.

184. "Europe's Lesson in War Relief: American Red Cross through Military Department is Organizing Base Hospital Units and Field Columns," *ARC Magazine* 11, no. 4 (April 1916): 111–14.

Disclosure. The author has no relevant financial interest or affiliations with any commercial interests related to the subjects discussed within this article.

MARIAN MOSER JONES, PHD, MPH
Associate Professor and Director of Graduate Studies
Department of Family Science
University of Maryland School of Public Health
1142BB School of Public Health Building
College Park, MD 20742

The Nurses No-One Remembers: Looking for Spanish Nurses in Accounts of the Spanish Civil War (1936–1939)

SIOBAN NELSON
University of Toronto, Canada

PAOLA GALBANY-ESTRAGUÉS
University of Vic-Central University of Catalonia, Spain

GLORIA GALLEGO-CAMINERO
University of Balearic Islands, Spain

Abstract. Accounts of Spanish nursing and nurses during the Spanish Civil War (1936–1939) that appear in the memoirs and correspondence of International Brigade volunteers, and are subsequently repeated in the secondary literature on the war, give little indication of existence of trained nurses in country. We set out to examine this apparent erasure of the long tradition of skilled nursing in Spain and the invisibility of thousands of Spanish nurses engaged in the war effort. We ask two questions: How can we understand the narrative thrust of the international volunteer accounts and subsequent historiography? And what was the state of nursing in Spain on the Republican side during the war as presented by Spanish participants and historians? We put the case that the narrative erasure of Spanish professional nursing prior to the Civil War was the result of the politicization of nursing under the Second Republic, its repression and reengineering under the Franco dictatorship, and the subsequent national policy of "oblivion" or forgetting that dominated the country during the transition to democracy. This policy silenced the stories of veteran nurses and prevented an examination of the impact of the Civil War on the Spanish nursing profession.

Nursing History Review 28 (2020): 63–92. A Publication of the American Association for the History of Nursing. Copyright © 2020 Springer Publishing Company.
http://dx.doi.org/10.1891/1062-8061.28.63

"We are the nurses no-one remembers" lamented Ana Pibernat in her memoirs of the Spanish Civil War (SCW; 1936–1939).[1] The conventional view of nursing in Spain during the war, espoused by the International Brigade (IB) volunteers in their memoirs and correspondence, and repeated in the secondary literature on the war all support Pibernat's contention, giving little indication of the existence of trained nurses in the country and even going so far as to declare them non existent. This observation, and its constant repetition, caused us to wonder at the apparent erasure of the centuries of skilled nursing in Spain and the thousands of Spanish nurses engaged in the war effort on both sides.

In what follows we examine these primary and secondary accounts of Spanish nursing by English language authors and attempt to understand the narrative construction of nursing in Spain. At the same time, we provide a counter-narrative of Spanish nursing on the Republican side, based on Spanish primary sources and secondary scholarship on the topic. We ask two questions: How can we understand the narrative thrust of the international volunteer accounts and subsequent historiography? And what was the state of nursing in Spain on the Republican side during the war as presented by Spanish participants and historians?

The story of *La Guerra Civil Española*, the SCW remains a deeply wounding and divisive episode in Spanish history. The war began on the 17th of July 1936 with a failed military coup d'etat in the Spanish Protectorate in Morocco. It ended with the defeat of Republican (Government) forces 3 years later, tearing apart regions, institutions, communities, and families. No part of society was immune from the brutal upheaval and deep divisions it left in its wake.[2] Moreover, under the *Dictadura* of the victorious Francisco Franco, who led the country from the end of the war in 1939 till his death in 1975, it was forbidden to publish on and dangerous to speak openly about the events of those 3 years. During the transition to democracy in the post-Franco era, the Pact of Oblivion continued this imposed silence under the goal of national reconciliation. Thus, in Spain, the question of the war, its atrocities, and its aftermath remains one of great contention as the nation continues to deal with the challenge of remembering.[3]

The Second Spanish Republic (1931–1939) was a progressive government with a radical agenda that sought the reform of the country's most powerful institutions. It implemented major changes to the military and abolished many of the long-held privileges of the Catholic Church.[4] It promoted regional autonomy and agrarian reform, introduced equal rights for women, including the right to education, civil marriage, consensual divorce, maternity insurance, and even abortion (although the latter was never implemented).[5] It also initiated major reforms to public health, nursing education, and nursing services.

This broad program of reform was seen as a direct threat to the nation's powerful conservative forces: the landlords, the Catholic Church, and the army, all of which coalesced around the nationalist or rebel forces opposing the Republic.[6]

In the mid-1930s, Europe was gripped by a series of crises as radical and reformist governments fell to right-wing and fascist regimes. In Portugal, Italy, and Germany, right-wing governments imprisoned their critics, attacked democratic institutions and increased surveillance of leftists and Jewish citizens. Meanwhile, France's fragile leftist government had to deal with powerful right-wing forces, while the British government pursued its disastrous appeasement stance against Hitler. Both countries failed to support the embattled Republic of Spain. Beyond Europe, the militaristic regime of Japan was growing in strength, and the home-grown fascist movements in the United States and elsewhere were becoming emboldened. Fear of Bolshevism set the tone for international relations in the west and the fact that the Spanish government's only allies were the communist governments of Mexico and Russia heightened the diplomatic tensions. For pro-democratic and leftist individuals, it was apparent that the world was on the brink of a descent into fascism.

Despite the recalcitrant positions taken by their respective governments, pro-democratic and leftist organizations and trade unionists around the world enthusiastically recruited volunteers for Spain to defend the embattled Republican government from the attack of Nationalist forces. The volunteers responded in their thousands,[7] and the resulting IB threw its weight behind the coalition of anarchists, communists, and republican forces that constituted the Republican side. Overall approximately 700,000 people fought on the Republican side in the war. This figure includes the 35,000 foreigners from 53 countries who served in the IBs, among whom were hundreds of nurses.

The international nurses who went to Spain, with only a handful of exceptions, volunteered on the side of the Republic. It is not possible to determine exactly how many nurses came. The highest estimate comes from Oscar Telge, a Bulgarian major who was head of the International Health Service. In 1937, he notes there were "more than 240 doctors, 600 nurses (men and women) and 650 orderlies working for our Organization."[8] A more conservative number of 203 appeared on a 1937 military document listing source countries but no names of individual nurses.[9]

As part of a separate and on-going project that has been published in Spanish and presented in English, we undertook to learn more about the nurses who volunteered in Spain. We examined the vast primary and secondary literature on the SCW and the IBs looking for references to nurses, nursing, or hospital work.[10] Our review included English, Spanish, French, Catalan, Italian, and Portuguese literature between 1936 and 2018 inclusive. We identified references to nursing in the biographies, memoirs,[11] journalist correspondence, and testimonies from wounded combatants and from health professionals and workers, such as physicians, orderlies, ambulance drivers, and laboratory technicians.[12]

From our research, we believe the actual number is closer to Telge's estimate. To date, we have identified 342 nurses from 40 countries out of what we believe to be the approximately 600 nurses who came to Spain to volunteer during the War. About half of these nurses were English speaking, many of whom come from leftist and or Jewish background. Of the remainder, women came for all across Europe, from Iceland to Austria, again a significant number appear to have been Jewish. We plan to publish these results in a separate paper.

One of the surprising findings of our review of the primary and secondary source material on nursing during the Civil War was the existence of a consistent series of observations on the state of Spanish hospitals and Spanish nurses. These observations typically comment on the absence of a nursing profession in Spain. As there are limited sources that describe Spanish nurses or the state of Spanish nursing, those sources that do exist have perhaps received undue authority in subsequent scholarship on the war. For instance, one high-profile observation comes from the recollections of volunteer soldier Eric Blair (George Orwell):

> Apparently there was no supply of trained nurses in Spain, perhaps because before the war this work was done chiefly by nuns. I have no complaint against the Spanish nurses, they always treated me with the greatest kindness, but there is no doubt they were terribly ignorant.[13]

Orwell's observation echoes that of other volunteers who claimed that Spain had no real trained nurses. Annie Murray, Scottish volunteer nurse later recalled: "They used nuns. So, these little Spanish girls only had about 3 months training. But they were very keen and very good for the time they had trained."[14]

The most well-known work on IB nurses and nursing in Spain during the war is that of British historian Angela Jackson whose pioneering work on British women volunteers and her subsequent biography of English IB nurse, Patience Darton, were published in 2002 and 2014 respectively. Over her long and active life, Darton had become the authoritative voice on the standard of Spanish nursing, medicine, and hospitals:

> Standards of Hygiene and asepsis were low at that time in Spain, and there was no tradition of nursing training comparable with that in Britain . . . nursing care of the patients was generally carried out by other family members or by nuns.[15]

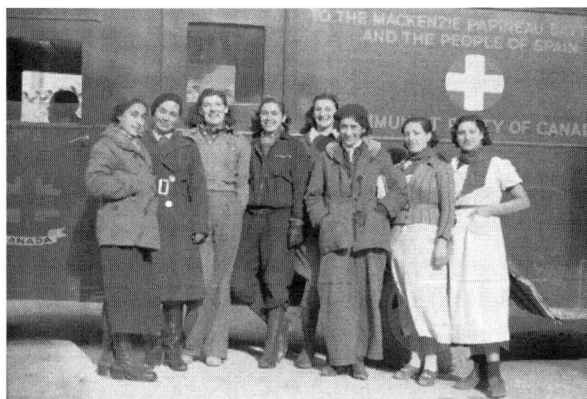

Figure 1. American nurses in front of an ambulance donated by the Communist Party of Canada. Left to right: Rose Weiner, Leonora (Nora) Temple, Toby Jensky, Anna Taft, Sara Goldblatt, Selma Chadwich, and Andrea y Leoncia (Spanish girls). Probably Alcorisa (Teruel). Aragon Front, January 1938. Unknown photographer (Reprinted permission, Archives of Marx Memorial Library, London).

IB nurse Ruth Wilson Epstein's Radio Madrid Broadcast to the United States on January 10, 1938, describes the challenging situation that faced the Republican side and the Brigadist hospitals. She speaks about the improvised classroom she established for local illiterate chicas who she taught rudimentary nursing in what she calls the region's "first nursing school"[1] (see Figure 1).

Jackson reports on Darton's observations concerning the modesty of the Spanish nurses, how they were unwilling to wash male patients[17] and the fact that "it wasn't a good thing for a Spanish girl of any sort, to go and work in a hospital with men." She presents Darton's picture of backward squalid hospitals and ignorant Spanish doctors and nurses (such as the physician who tried to prevent Darton from washing her British typhoid patient).[18] Given the observations found in eyewitness accounts, it is no surprise that the secondary literature builds on this theme. In 1986 Fryth describes the situation as the following:

> There were some very good hospitals, especially in Republican-held Madrid and Barcelona, but nursing services were scanty; hospitals were run by nuns and patients were generally nursed by their own families, who moved in with them, as in the days of the Crimean War. Standards of hygiene, as the British nurses were to discover, were sometimes horrifying.[19]

And in the repetition, the myth grows stronger. In 2013, Linda Palfreeman, in her book *Aristocrats, Adventurers and Ambulances* describes nurses as a rarity in Spain with care relying on family members.

At the outbreak of Civil War Spain could boast some excellent hospitals, especially in Madrid and Barcelona, but they were run by nuns and other assistants with very little professional training. Expert nursing care was rarity and patients had to be cared for by members of their own family.[20]

There is no question as to the validity of the observations and experiences of the eye witness accounts of nursing during the war. What is interesting, however, is the conclusion they draw from these observations, and secondly, how it is that they miss so much of the picture. The descriptions by volunteers and repeated by subsequent British historians on the lack of skill of Spanish nurses and the backwardness of Spanish hospitals were based on several assumptions: first that the nursing care of religious sisters or nuns was the equivalent of poor nursing. Second, that knowledge of hospital management and asepsis and hygiene were entirely lacking in the country. Third, that professional secular nursing did not exist in Spain. Let us take these three points in turn.

First, it is important to understand that the Republican or Government side of the Civil War was characterized by extreme anticlericalism (particularly in Barcelona and Andalusia). The Catholic Church was hostile to the secular reforms implemented by the Republic and was a key supporter of the Nationalist rebels. In this context, the Republican view of religious nurses was generally unsympathetic.

Moreover, the dismissal of nursing by religious nurses as antithetical to high-quality nursing is a common categorical error made by nursing and general historians alike. In fact, nursing by religious women and men has a long and distinguished history in Spain.[21] While not all religious orders were known for their commitment to nursing, nor for their leadership in running the best hospitals, the truly excellent hospitals in Madrid and Barcelona specifically referred to by Fryth and others were operated by nursing sisterhoods. Far from being backward, these institutions were the home base of many of the medical and surgical innovators.[22]

The major problem with the Spanish reliance on religious nurses was that the anti-clerical sentiments of the pro-government side of the conflict meant that the sisters overwhelmingly (but not entirely) abandoned their posts and fled to the nationalist side at the onset of the conflict.[23] Thus the standard of nursing care and hospital management observed by members of the IBs was Spanish nursing without a key element of its workforce—religious nurses. Brigadists drew their own conclusions from this observation deciding that Spanish nursing was backward and lacking in professionalism, a comparison that reflected well on British and American nurses.

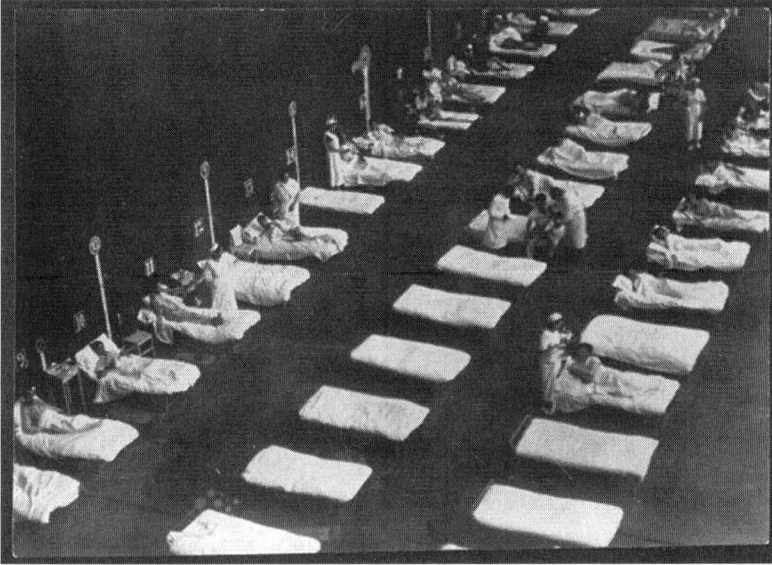

Figure 2. Wounded assisted by civilian nurses at the Provisional Blood Hospital installed on the Fronton of Recoletos by the Libertarian Athenian of Delicias of CNT (Workers National Confederation). Madrid, 1936–1937. Reprinted with the permission of the National Library of Spain.

The second issue concerning poor hospital management and lack of hygiene or knowledge of asepsis arises from a similar lack of contextual understanding. It was not until later in the war that Republican forces possessed a formal medical unit. The military (with few exceptions) supported the Nationalist cause and the medical organization and equipment went to that side, as did religious nurses fleeing anti-clerical forces. Therefore the Republicans, including the volunteer brigades, took some time to put into place their medical infrastructure, both personnel, and equipment (see Figure 2).

There are many accounts of the appalling conditions facing the medical and nursing volunteers when they arrived, whether it was setting up a hospital in a filthy barn, or a sports stadium taking over an overwhelmed improvised hospital or one captured from the nationalist side. In each instance, these stories become a vehicle to tell of the scrubbing and hard work, the improvising with makeshift or antiquated equipment, the bartering for food and water from the local mayor and so forth. In the case of the hospital changing hands, there were often outraged stories of infections and filth, often at the hands of sisters.[24]

These Republican stories against religious nurses warrant scrutiny. The evidence of callous and poor nursing by religious nurses witnessed by volunteers is very hard to interpret. It is difficult to know whether the sisters were in fact nurses, or merely volunteers. Thus, the lack of knowledge concerning hygiene or wound care may represent unskilled nursing rather than religious nursing. Without more information, the assumptions drawn by the IB volunteers may have merely been confirming their biases rather than offering conclusive evidence on the backwardness of Spanish nursing and hospital care. One counter story comes from the biographical account of Manuel Álvarez who as a youth was wounded in the war. He later searched for the Canadian volunteer who saved his life. His first-person account is in stark contrast to that offered by so many IB accounts.

Since 1938, whether as a patient or as a visitor, I have known many hospitals around the world, but I still consider the one in Vilanova y la Geltrú the best of all, it was governed by nuns, all of them competent. In the advent of the Revolution, they replaced their habits with nurse uniforms, civil people had replaced the nuns in the administration of the hospital, but in practice, the organization of the hospital continued to unfold very much like a convent, with the mother superior as Director of the institution, the assistance was unbeatable, the nutrition excellent, the atmosphere was saturated by the pious courtesy of those nuns, the whole building was magnificent: high ceiling rooms, large windows opening into a flowered garden.[25]

The first-person accounts of appalling conditions underline the vital role of volunteer nurses in the IB narratives, serving a critical propaganda function back home. In these foreigners' narratives for foreign readers, Spanish nurses are relegated to minor supportive roles of wonderful but ignorant local "chicas" or girls, whom IB nurses trained in basic nursing over the course of the conflict. In one of the few papers that looks at Spanish nurses and nursing during the Civil War, Isabel Anton-Solanas, Ann Wakefield, and Christine Hallett[26] undertook an analysis of the published accounts by IB nurses to explore the relationship between Spanish and IB nurses. They found sparse evidence of contact between IB nurses and trained Spanish nurses. Anton-Solanas and colleagues were primarily interested in whether the IB nurses had a lasting impact on Spanish nursing, but it is not a question they are able to resolve. In a somewhat solipsistic argument they claim that: "the fact that the international nurses openly acknowledged both the general evolution of Spanish nursing and the personal development of the Spanish women they had trained reveals a qualitative change in nursing services as the war evolved." They conclude that, despite the lack of supportive evidence, "the IB played their part in shaping and advancing Spanish nursing through their work and example."[27]

We fundamentally diverge from the arguments of Anton-Solanas and colleagues. Although we agree that the IB nurses infrequently encountered skilled Spanish nurses, we disagree as to the conclusions that may be drawn from this fact. The IB forces of 35,000 constituted only approximately 5% of the forces fighting on the Republic side during the war. That leaves 95% of the Republican forces and 100% of the rebel or Francoist forces who were served by Spanish medical and nursing teams. Furthermore, the cities, towns, and villages of Spain continued to require the care of doctors, *practicantes*, nurses, and midwives and, amid the desperation and chaos of war, that care continued as best it could.[28] In order to examine the story of Spanish nursing missing from the first person and secondary accounts of international volunteers, we will look at Spanish nursing in three parts: before the Civil War, during the war, and its aftermath.

Part One: Spanish Nursing Before the Civil War

It can be safely assumed foreign nurses knew little of the system of training, different types of licenses and programs that existed within Spain, nor did they understand the complex role of male and female nursing orders in the country (see Table 1, Official designations of nurses in Spain). Spanish nursing wasa particular mixture of highly skilled and professional religious and secular nurses, with state-based oversight for licensure that had been in place for centuries.[29]

In fact, Spain had conducted programs of education and training overseen by the national government since the 16th century, along with national examinations of men and women nurses of the different categories (midwives, bleeders, *practicantes*, and nurses). The *practicante* was a 19th-century initiative and can be best described as a medical assistant with a highly independent practice; these individuals tended to be male. Carmen Domínguez-Alcón identified at least 67 manuals of instruction on nursing care in Spanish were published in the 19th century[30] with a further 59 instruction manuals were published between 1900 and 1936.[31] The training of *practicantes* and midwives was continuously and officially regulated in Spain since 1857 with the implementation of the *Moyano Law*, which regulated education across the country, the law that oversaw the modernization of the Spanish education system in the mid-19th century. Even after the SCW, they were still appointed to villages and cities as municipal employees with an obligation to provide free of services to the poor.[32]

TABLE 1. Brief History of Nursing Licensing in Spain XIX to the Present Day

Designation	Official Rules
Matrona (Midwife) *Practicante* (Practitioner)	Both designations appear in the Moyano Law, or Law of Public Instruction edict (1857). This law replaced previous regulations concerning programs and exams for midwives, minor surgeons, or "bloodletters," and so forth. It introduced a 2 year program of four semesters in authorized centers with exams overseen by medical schools. Subsequent official decrees continued to regulate the studies and practice of these professions in 1861, 1888, and 1904.
Enfermera (Nurse)	Introduced in 1915 as an official designation in line with midwives and *practicantes.* Included religious and secular nurses.
ATS (Technical Health Assistant)	Decree of 4th December 1953, (BOE of 29th of December 1953) The decree brought together former midwives, *practicantes,* and nurses under a single designation: Technical Health Assistant. 3 years of study. Graduates could continue their studies in midwifery and other specialties. Membership of the College of Nursing required to work as a nurse.
Diplomado en enfermería (Diploma in Nursing)	On July 23, 1977 (BOE of August 22, 1977), the Technical Health Assistant schools were transformed into university schools of nursing. The new designation was Diploma in Nursing (3 years study). Applicants to Nursing required the same requirements for University admission as other studies (medicine, architecture, pharmacy, etc.).

(Continued)

TABLE 1. Brief History of Nursing Licensing in Spain XIX to the Present Day *(Continued)*

Designation	Official Rules
Técnico en Cuidados Auxiliares de Enfermería (Technician in auxiliary nursing care)	Commencing in 1996 auxiliary nurses were formalized in Spain. These programs are not university based and do not lead to enrollment in the Professionals Associations of Nurses (*colegios profesionales de enfermería*) in each capital of province. The *Auxiliares de enfermería* support the work of the diplomate College nurses.
Grado en enfermería (Nursing Graduate)	From 2009, degree entry to practice in Spain. The *Grado en enfermería* entails 4 years of study in conformity with nursing programs in other European countries.

Note. Registration with the regional college or professional association (colegios provinciales de enfermeria) was compulsory to work as a nurse. Religious nurses were not required under law to qualify in the smae manner until 1953, although many in fact conducted nursing schools and completed the same programs of study.

Religious nurses did not tend to undertake training as *practicantes* and were forbidden until the mid-20th century to be involved in midwifery practice. Therefore their training tended to take place in their hospitals and, before 1915, in Italy. When training for nurses was regularized, along with midwives and *practicantes* in 1915, religious sisters undertook the same preparation as secular nurses.

Over the course of the 19th and 20th century, Spanish nursing continued to evolve its licensure processes and increased the numbers of non-religious nursing schools in the country. Although there is no single data source for the number of trained nurses in Spain prior to the war, one can get a sense of how many trained secular nurses there were at the outbreak of the war looking at the various training programs and numbers of graduates sitting national examinations. 18 years before the Civil War, in 1917, in addition to long-established schools, the Spanish Red Cross, or *Cruz Roja*, established 32 schools of nurses in Spain. The Schools developed their own manuals for theoretical and practical courses. In 1921 the *Cruz Roja* had 30 training centers of voluntary nurses unpaid, who had trained to 729 volunteers nurses.[33] (See Table 2 for a summary of the Leading Nursing Schools in Spain prior to the Civil War.)

By 1931 the number of women receiving instruction from *Cruz Roja* was 526.[34] That same year, 366 nurses took the first State examination of nurses at

TABLE 2. Principal Schools of Nursing before the Spanish Civil War

Active	City	Name	Observations
1896–1936	Madrid	*Escuela Santa Isabel de Hungría en el Instituto de Terapéutica Operatoria* (St. Isabel of Hungary School at the Institute of Surgical Therapy). The candidates lived in and were subject to strict oversight over the 3 years.	Destroyed during the SCW
1914–up to day	Madrid	*Escuela de enfermeras de la Cruz Roja* (Red Cross Nurses School). They taught both registered and volunteer (unpaid) nurses.	In 1921 there were *Damas Enfermeras de La Cruz Roja* (Ladies Nurses of the Red Cross) in all Spanish provinces
1917–2010	Barcelona	*Escola Universitària d'Infermeria Santa Madrona* (Nursing School St. Madrona).	Initially a 2-year program (161 students)
1919–1923	Barcelona	*Escola Especial d'Infermeres Auxiliars de la Medicina,* established by the regional government.	2 years. Closed during the Primo de Rivera Dictatorship
1924- to today	Madrid	*Escuela Nacional de Sanidad* (National Health School)	Established links with the Rockefeller Foundation, (fellowships for 14 nurses and a midwife between 1931 and 1936)
1929–to today	Santander	*Escuela de Enfermería de la Casa de Salud de Valdecilla* (School of Nursing of Valdecilla)	2 years. The students lived at the school.
1931–1936	Barcelona	*Escola d'Infermeres de la Generalitat de Catalunya* (School of Nursing of the Government of Catalonia, Spain)	2 years. The students lived at the school.

the Faculty of Medicine in Madrid. In 1934 the Visiting Nurses Professional Association, presided over by Mercedes Milá Molla, had 109 members.[35] At the end of November 1936, the number of nurses in the official College of Nurses of Catalonia, a region of Spain, was approaching five hundred. Between 1929 and 1936, 16,366 students in Catalonia applied to have their qualifications recognized. These included the three categories of nurse—nurses, *practicantes*, and midwives. In all 4,411 licenses were issued: 3,014 *practicantes*, midwives 721, and 676 nurses.[36] In addition to these formally licensed nurses under the Republic's new national provisions for title recognition, there was also an unknown number of nursing professionals who were covered under the Moyano Law (1857), which was still in effect for all three categories of nurse who had held their title since 1915.

By the 1930s, these modern nursing programs included instruction on public health nursing. Spain, like many countries around the world, was influenced by the rise of the American model of the public health nurse whose main role was to work with communities and families.[37] This new nurse was an educator and a change agent. Nurses on the left in the United States, such as Lavinia Dock and Lilian Wald and their colleagues in the settlement movement, set out to build supportive communities and promote health among the poorest and most vulnerable members of society. This early 20th-century movement, energized by the end of World War I and the influenza pandemic, was still gaining momentum in the United States and Canada in the 1930s and the nursing leadership in the United States, with the support of the Rockefeller Foundation, saw it as a key advance for both society, in terms of addressing the twin ills of ignorance and poverty, and for the nursing profession, as it provided an autonomous and authoritative community role for nurses independent of medical supervision and hospital hierarchies.

Nursing schools in Spain followed medical schools in the implementation of training programs for well-educated nurses with a strong foundation in public health, health education, and disease prevention. This was the pattern in the United States and Canada, no less than in Spain, and by the mid-1930s the numbers of training centers for nurses run by the *Cruz Roja* or by universities attached to medical schools had multiplied. At the same time, the older nursing schools based at the hospitals conducted by religious nurses continued to educate nurses who could qualify to meet the national requirements for credential recognition as trained nurses. As in other countries, there was a range of quality in such programs from the country's best and most innovative hospitals, to those with poorer standards of care.

So, despite the lack of precise numbers on trained nurses in Spain before the war, we can be confident that there were many thousands of secular nurses who were both trained and held the authorized title of nurse, *practicante*, or midwife. We can also say with certainty is that neither the Nationalist nor the Republican side had sufficient nurses, secular or religious, to meet demand at the beginning of the war.

Part 2: Spanish Nursing During the War

Although nursing in Spain had been evolving and progressing in line with peer countries during the first three decades of the 20th century, all of this was to come to an abrupt end with the commencement of the Civil War. As government and rebel forces split the country along battle lines, the lives of religious nurses came under threat in government-held territory and many fled to nationalist held regions. This alone would have constituted a major catastrophe for the provision of hospital care in the country but it was only the beginning. It was impossible to fill the gap made by the departure of religious nurses with fully trained secular nurses. Even before the war there had been insufficient nurses to meet national needs and the ambitious health program of the government had already deployed many nurses to its short-lived community programs. Gauging the number of nurses during the war on both sides is a challenge. However, in the Nationalist or Francoist zone, we have an idea of the overall number of nurses as the war progressed as a result of the issuance, in May 1938, of identity documents for 12,307 nurses and nurse assistants.[38] On the Republican side, we need to rely on first-person accounts such as those of Gaston Levale, referring to Barcelona, who wrote: "There were 1,000 doctors, 3,200 nurses, 330 midwives and six hundred dentists, working well and imaginatively."[39]

The chaos and disruption of Civil War meant that there was a desperate shortage of trained nurses. Both sides responded to this situation by the creation of short specific programs for war nurses. On the Republican side, a system of nurse training was established through trade unions and women organizations.[40] On the Nationalist side, they prepared military nurses, as Phalanx or the so-called *Margaritas*. The *Cruz Roja* trained nurses on both sides of the conflict[41] (see Figures 3 and 4). Martin and Ordonez describe how politically affiliated models of nursing burgeoned during the war, identifying nursing work as an opportunity for women to engage in the political life of the war.

Different models of nursing coexisted on the Republican side oriented by the political values, such as those of the Anarchists, of Trotskyists, of communists and of liberals and even on the Francoist side, included simultaneously royalist and Falangist women and others who supported traditionalist ideologies.[42]

Over the course of the war three types of Spanish nurses were introduced: qualified nurses (or the equivalent as registration is not a term used in Spain),

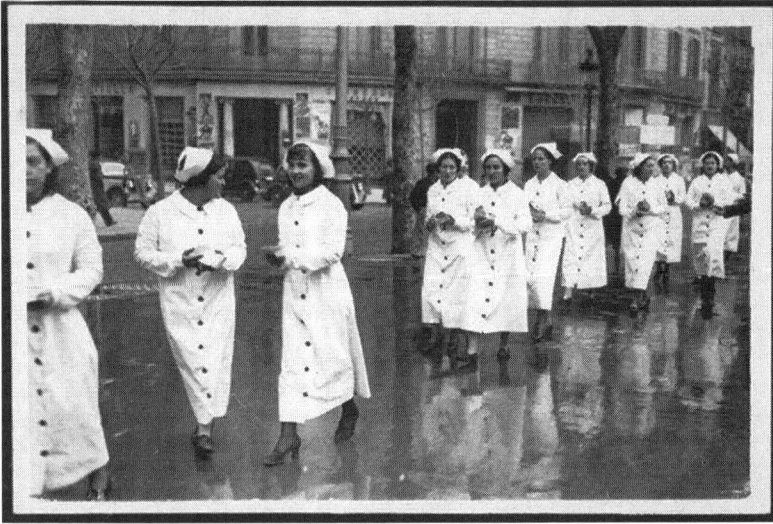

Figure 3. A row of nursing students walking down a street. Probably in Calle Cortes (Today Gran Vía de les Corts Catalanes, 690). Calle Cortes housed a training center for *infermeras de guerra* of the Free Women of the FAI (Iberian Anarchist Federation). Barcelona, probably winter 1936–37. Photographer Pau Lluis Torrents (National Library of Spain, with permission of the Torrens family).

nurses with "titles of war," or *infermeras de Guerra,* who were graduates of union or women organization's short training programs (a few months), and nursing aides or assistants (no training). Occasionally, individuals—Spanish and foreign—without any preparation in nursing volunteered to help the wounded and sick as nursing assistants. On the Republican side, writers, artists, photographers worked as these type of nurses with the IBs.[43] On both sides, Spanish nurses who wished to have their qualifications upgraded from *infermera de guerra* to nurse, underwent further training programs and additional examinations in order to receive their official nursing certification.[44]

   An important collection of essays, *Enfermeras de Guerra,* edited by Anna Ramio and Carmen Torres, published in Spanish in 2015, sets out the war experience of thirteen Spanish nurses.[45] The work is divided into sections distinguishing between nurses who qualified before the war, nurses who underwent training during the war as *infermeras de guerra,* and did not continue as nurses at the end of hostilities, and nurses who commenced training during the war and continued in the profession afterward. The women were interviewed by a team of researchers as part of an extensive oral history project on nursing during the war. The research highlights the diversity of backgrounds,

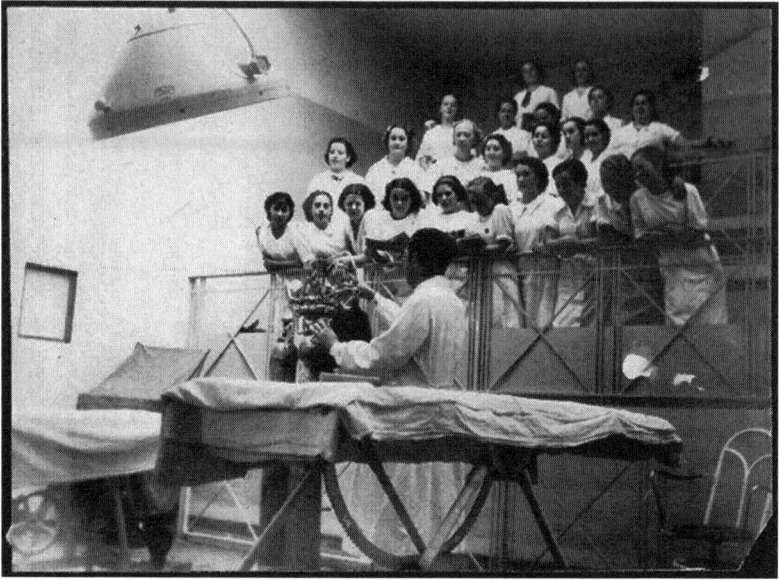

Figure 4. A group of 26 students attending a practice class. Probably Barcelona. 1936–1939. Reprinted with the permission of the National Library of Spain.

religious and political affiliations, education pathways, and subsequent lives of these women. It also highlights the wide range of work they undertook during the war, the diversity of training and mentorship provided and how the experience impacted their future. The women interviewed worked in major hospitals in Barcelona, in rural areas, in maternal and infant care, surgery, tuberculosis, anesthetics, and multiple other areas of practice.

Some of the most important insights and recollections provided by Ramio, Torres, and colleagues deal with the transitions at the beginning and end of the war. These nurses describe the extraordinary effort to fill the gap made by the loss of so many religious nurses with the commencement of hostilities, and the vital contribution of those nuns (in civilian dress and at great risk) who remained in Republican-controlled areas in training the vast numbers of women who responded to the radio call for volunteers to staff the hospitals and clinics (see Figure 5).

Much was accomplished in those first months of the war when the Republican side needed to establish an entire military medical infrastructure of advanced and rearguard hospitals. The lack of pre-existing infrastructure led to creative innovations, such as the mobile operating clinics (see Figure 6), and the mobile blood service that the Republican medical teams became famous

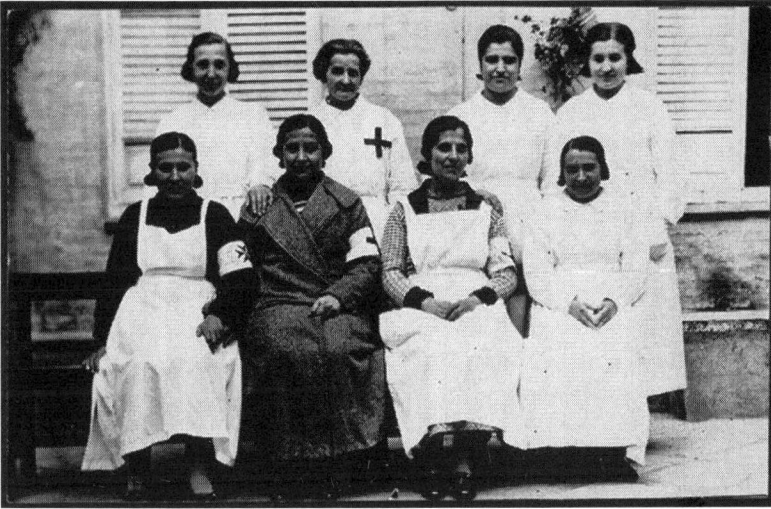

Figure 5.   Group of eight women. Text on the back of the photograph translates as: *Old Carmelite nuns, today nurses of the hospital of Andújar*. Andújar (Jaén, Spain) 1936–1939. Reprinted with the permission of the National Library of Spain.

for during the war, and were widely imitated in World War II. The transition at the end of the war, when the Nationalist forces took control, was another chaotic time. Although Spanish doctors and nurses were among the thousands of exiles who departed under fire to France, many others held to their posts and continued to work as the religious nurses took back control of the health institutions across the country.

Further insight into the world of nursing during the war can be found in *Shining Beacons in the Darkness: Memories of Saving Lives during the Spanish Civil War in Catalunya*.[46] Published in 2013 in Catalan and English by *Del Memorial Democratic Generalitat de Catalunya*, this work is combination of first person and scholarly accounts of the healthcare and aid by doctors, nurses and emergency workers, general citizens and foreigners during the war, the very great dangers they faced both not only from the war directly, but from their Republican colleagues should their loyalties ever be suspect.

One ugly challenge of Civil War that affected the availability of skilled nurses and doctors was the difficulty in distinguishing enemy from friend. The catastrophic shortage of nurses on both sides[47] was exacerbated by the debug-ging of "politically suspect" civilian nurses. *Depuradas* was the term for nurses and doctors in the Francoist area who were unable to practice because they were considered politically suspect. On both sides of the conflict, there were

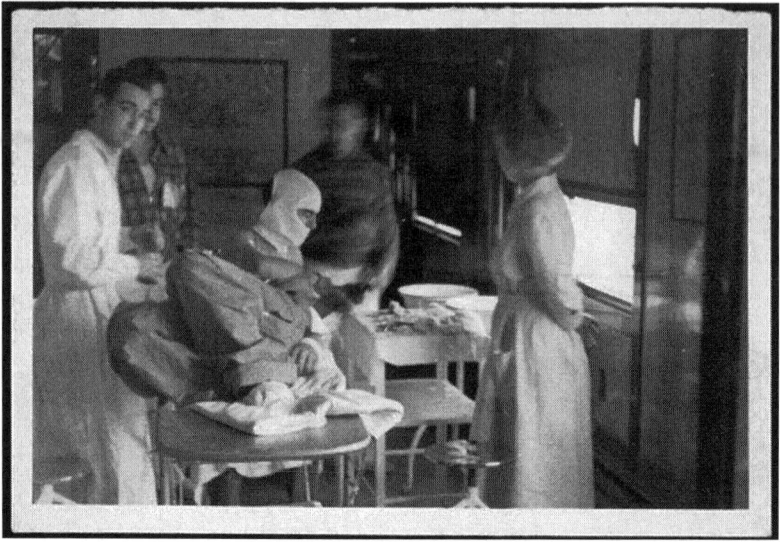

Figure 6. Inside one of the treatment rooms where surgeons and nurses attended to the wounded on a hospital train. Unknown place, probably 1936–1937. Photographer Centelles. Reprinted with the permission of the National Library of Spain.

harsh measures for spies or fifth columnists, and this vigilance and paranoia played out in every workplace, community, and sector throughout the country. In fact, nurses suffered greatly in this climate of suspicion because of their access to the battlefront and to wounded men who may inadvertently reveal classified information. On both sides, courses for nurses were introduced that included ideological indoctrination and nurses had to demonstrate political correctness to be permitted to work.

Republican nurse Ana Pibernat Caner's memoir is rich in its detail of front line service and typhoid fever nursing.[48] Pibernat was a graduate of the nursing program in Girona where she completed primary studies and 2 years of nursing, achieving her license just before the commencement of the SCW. She was one of the growing number of graduates from newly established schools of nursing under the Second Republic, which were committed to public health and in which the nursing profession was considered a major resource in their programs for improvement of health in the population, with nurse-led community health programs.[49]

During the war, Pibernat volunteered to the front line hospital located in a train tunnel between Flix and Asco (Tarragona). She was also at the hospital at Valls during the typhoid epidemic and at the end of the war participated in the evacuation of the wounded during the retreat: "from hospital to hospital" to Figueras at the French border.[50] Trinidad Gallego Prieto, like Pibernat, was an experienced and qualified nurse who had worked under the Second Republic before the war.[51] Gallego was also a midwife and she had been actively involved in implementing the Republican government's reforms of maternal care which shifted the model from punitive to supportive care for unmarried pregnant women and new mothers. During the war, she was the head nurse at the Hospital Clinico de San Carlos de Madrid which attended wounded military and civilian patients.

Only one nurse of the thirteen profiled in the collection by Ramio and Torres matches the profile of the willing "chicas" described in so many of the recollections of the brigadists. Maria Sans Moyer, an *infermera de guerra*, was stationed at a brigadist hospital and was trained by a British IB nurse.[52] She spent the war entirely with brigadist forces and was a veteran of the Battle of Ebro. In fact, Maria Sans Moyer is believed to be the inspiration for Hemmingway's character Maria, in *For Whom the Bell Tolls*.[53]

If Sans Moyer exemplifies the nurse who is the subject of so many first-person accounts by IB volunteers, Trinidad Gallego Prieto and Ana Pabernat typify the new nurse of the Second Republic seldom encountered by the volunteers. These nurses were well educated and professional, had a strong commitment to justice and saw the important role the nursing profession had to play in the reform and democratization of society.[54] They also typify the kind of nurse that the dictatorship was determined to eradicate. The defeated Second Republic had aligned a feminist reform agenda and the public health agenda. They had recognized the potential for women to play a major part in their social reform program both as leaders and workers, and nursing and midwifery were key to the implementation of these reforms which directly affected women and children. Following the war, the public health programs that had been central to the Republic's reform platform were abandoned.

Part 3: The Aftermath

As the defeat of the Government forces became more certain, the IBs formally withdrew. This was a terrible time for the volunteers and for the nursing and medical teams there was the additional trauma of abandoning not just colleagues and comrades, but patients. And as Europe descended into World War II many of the volunteers found the door home closed behind them. The false documents and illegal border crossings, which had been necessary to enter Spain, made the return journey particularly difficult. For those volunteers from countries with fascist Governments, there could be no return for "red" volunteers. This was especially the case for those of Jewish ancestry.[55]

For the defeated Spanish Republicans, the situation was also desperate. Following the exodus under fire of tens of thousands of Spanish refugees to France. Internment camps were established by the French government. These camps had appalling conditions and accompanying high death rates from disease and exposure. Foreigners and Jews were handed over to the Gestapo following the German invasion of France in 1940. This was the fate of Austrian IB volunteer Auguste Guttman, a nurse veteran of the Great War. Guttman had arrived in Spain in August 1937 and remained until the evacuation of Catalonia, a Republican stronghold, working at the Hospital at Villaneuva de la Jara. She is believed to have died in Auschwitz.[56] The exiled nurse Aurora Fernández also left testimony of this hardship and human tragedy in her unpublished memoirs.[57]

Those who remained in Spain risked fierce retribution. In the violence and recrimination that followed the Civil War, the experience of these doctors and nurses very much depended on their political profile during the war (and that of their families), and on luck. For some, the transition was very challenging but in the end they simply kept working, for others there was no possibility of continuing their work as doctors and nurses. Republicans who survived torture and imprisonment were forbidden to practice in their professions and many were forced into exile.[58] Republican nurses faced humiliation as a "red" women, along with the suspension of their nursing licenses under the Francoist regime.[59] The young Spanish women who had been trained by the IB nurses at improvised auxiliary nursing units at the hospitals were accused of collaboration with the reds. They were prohibited from taking advantage of the knowledge and skills they had learned as auxiliaries of foreign nurses, unable to work as nurses after the war.

In February 1939 Ana Pibernat, along with four other nurses and an abandoned child crossed the Pyrenees. She returned to Spain in 1940 but was forced to escape from her village to avoid violent retribution. Her nursing license was invalidated under Franco and she was unable to gain permission to take the new exam as several of her family members were in prison during the early years of Franco's dictatorship. Trinidad Gallego was imprisoned at the end of the war, along with her mother and grandmother, and in and out of jail a total of sixteen times. Each time she provided nursing and midwifery care to the women and children in the jails. It was not until 1969, 30 years after the war, that she was once again permitted to work as a nurse and midwife.[60] *Infermera de guerra*, Maria Sans Moyer also fell victim to the persecution of "reds" that followed the war. With her father and brother in prison and her sister in Argentina, San Moyer was forbidden from continuing in nursing.[61]

Unlike the boost in professional standing for nursing that took place post World War II in the Allied nations, nothing remained of the high levels of nursing skill and innovation practiced by the international nurses and their colleagues in Spain. In fact, professional nursing took a backward step following the defeat of the Republic.[62] During the postwar period jobs for nurses in hospitals, once again under the control of the Catholic Church and managed by religious sisterhoods, were preferentially granted to the minimally trained *infermeras de guerra*, on the Pro-Franco side. In this way, many nurses with little education managed to enter the profession. At the same time curricula that paid attention to primary healthcare, public health or community care, or any specializations such as were advanced by nurses under the Second Republic, were abandoned for decades.[63]

Following the war, nurses who had qualified during the pre-war period were required to have their credentials reviewed, perhaps reexamined, and to obtain a certificate of good conduct.[64] And for the Republicans who remained or returned to Spain during the Franco years, many sacrificed the possibility of working as registered nurses, as they refused to undergo the humiliation of reexamination and "Social Service" compulsory for women aged 17 to 35 years. The latter was a means of control and immersion in the Francoist ideology and obligatory for women, the equivalent of national service for men, prior to applying for any official documentation such as a passport or driving license.

With the victory of conservative forces, the reformist agenda of the Republic was turned back and its nascent initiatives eradicated, along with the programs that supported contraception and gave women significant rights for divorce and custody of children. The professionalized, university educated, public health-focused professions of nursing and midwifery were considered suspect and antithetical to the values of the church and patristic state under Franco.

In the decades following the war, as the turmoil of transition and rebuilding hospitals and healthcare began, there was a clear need for significant reform of the system. Like the Republic before it, the Dictatura needed to modernize its systems and to improve the education and skill of the health workforce to meet the needs of 20th-century healthcare. Furthermore, because of the complexity of the postwar period which facilitated the integration of *infermeras de guerra*, on the victorious nationalist side, and excluded so many qualified nurses who had been in the Republican sector, the level of knowledge and skill among nurses was no longer standardized until 1953.

As Siles argues with respect to both Spain and Latin America, authoritarian or dictatorial regimes with their emphasis on conservative patriarchal values, result in diminished professional status for nursing.[65] Not only were republican or suspect nurses banned or forced to undergo ideological based training, but the profession itself became the target of social reengineering under Franco. In 1953, the dictatorship responded to the demands of hospital development and expansion to reform the education and professional standing of nurses. The previously distinct categories of nurses: midwives (*matronas*), *practicantes*, and nurses (*enfermeras*) were consolidated into a single program and certification process under a new title. In 1953, the titles of "nurse" (*enfermera*) and "midwife" (*matrona*) were downgraded to "Assistant Health Technician" (*Ayudante Técnico Sanitario*, ATS), a title that was highly unpopular with the majority of nurses and midwives and yet remained in place until 1977 after the death of Franco. Students of ATS were divided by gender. Female students attended training schools with mandatory boarding, and the curriculum was specifically oriented by gender to reflect the values of the patristic state.[66] The ATS program did succeed in raising the entry requirements from the postwar low and improved the level of preparedness of the hospital workforce. However, it also made clear that the sole aim of these new health workers was to be auxiliary to and a support for medicine.[67] Under the close direction of the Women's Section of the Falangist Party, the Church, and the medical profession, nursing education was stripped of all professionalizing sentiments and infused with the patristic values of the regime and devoted to subservience to medicine and the Catholic state.[68] Nursing had to wait until the death of Franco to reemerge as a full profession under the titles of nurse (*enfermera*) and midwife (*matrona*) once more. With the passing of the dictator, all nursing studies were instated at the University level as *Diplomados en Enfermeria* (Nursing Diplomates; See Table 1).

Conclusion

The scholarly renaissance in interest in the SCW in the 80s and 90s, particularly from British and American historians, led to a surge of publications on the topic of the war and the role of brigadists—men and women.

One of the casualties of this narrative was the story of Spanish nurses. The grim portrayals of the conditions of Spanish hospitals have been taken as reflective of the actual state of Spanish nursing, rather than the state of volunteer nursing in wartime. Such views have reified foreign expertise at the expense of their Spanish colleagues and shaped both the internal and the external view of the profession and healthcare in Spain prior to the war.

The story of nursing in Spain during the war is a complicated history that divides republican and nationalist sides. The Catholic Church had long played a central role in Spanish society and in the postwar period it regained a strong presence in education and healthcare. What the IB nurses and volunteers witnessed during the chaos of the Civil War was a profession sundered by pro and anti-clerical ideologies at war. The Civil War ruptured the profession with the losers the secular, university educated public health nursing movement which took some 50 years to recover.

Given this subsequent course of events, we argue, it is indeed worth understanding both the context and impact of the apparent absence of professional nursing and skilled nurses during the SCW by the very many writers from all over the world who have written on the war. It seems that Catalan nurse Ana Pibernat was correct when she lamented "We are the nurses no-one remembers."[69] Under Franco such remembering was forbidden. Under the Pact of Oblivion it was discouraged. Only now, as so many of the nurses are gone, are their stories beginning to surface and nursing under the Second Republic, that important period in Spanish nursing history, can become part of the narrative of nursing and of women in 20th-century Spain.

Notes

1. Ana Pibernat, "Ana Pibernat Caner. Mis Memorias," in *Memorias del Pueblo*, ed. Amparo Hurtado (Barcelona, Spain: RBA, 2004), 37–63.
2. The Franco dictatorship did not represent a homogeneous period. There were several stages: The first between 1939 and 1950, characterized by extreme repression and international isolation, the second between 1951 and 1965 characterized by greater international support, and the third between 1966 and 1975 (*Tardofranquismo*) characterized by economic development and opening. See Javier Tusell, "La Dictadura franquista," in *Historia de España*, ed. John Lynch, vol. XIX (Madrid, Spain: El País, 2007). For a general and classic text on the war, widely read both within Spain (although banned during the dictatorship) and throughout the world see Hugh Thomas, *The Spanish Civil War* (New York: Harper and Row, 1961), 616. About the civil war from broad perspective see Paul Preston, *The Spanish Civil War: Reaction, Revolution, and Revenge. Revised and Expanded Edition* (WW Norton & Company, New York, 2007); Raymond Carr, *The Spanish Tragedy: the Civil War in Perspective* (Phoenix Press, London, 2000). For Spanish literature see Julián Casanovas, "Sólo en España hubo guerra civil," *El País*, Madrid, July 17, 2011, http://elpais.com/diario/2011/07/17/domingo/1310874758_850215.html; Angel Viñas, *El Combate por la Historia. La República, la Guerra Civil, el Franquismo* (Barcelona, Spain: Pasado & Presente, 2012).

3. The Pacto de Olvido, or the Pact of Forgetting, in English was an agreement among the political parties to assist in the transition to democracy at the end of the dictatorship. Legally underpinned by the Spanish Amnesty Law of 1977 it prevents the prosecution of war crimes during the war or under Franco's rule. See Madeleine Davis, "Is Spain Recovering its Memory? Breaking the 'Pacto de Olvido," *Human Rights Quarterly* 27 (2005): 858–80.

4. Francisco José Romero Salvadó, "Killing the Dream: The Spanish Labyrinth Revisited, 1989–1939," in *Looking back at the Spanish Civil War. The International Brigade Memorial Trust, Len Crome Memorial Lectures, 2002–2010*, ed. Jim Jump (London, UK: Lawrence & Wishart, 2010), 48.

5. Martha A. Ackelsberg, *Free Women of Spain: Anarchism and the Struggle for the Emancipation of Women* (Edinburgh, Scotland: AK Press, 2005), 167; Mary Nash and Irene Cifuentes, *Rojas: Las Mujeres Republicanas en La Guerra Civil* (Madrid, Spain: Taurus Historia, 2006), 233–47.

6. Antony Beevor, *The Battle for Spain: The Spanish Civil War 1936–1939* (London, UK: Weidenfeld and Nicolson, 2006), 91.

7. The nationalities (with more than a thousand fighters) from the highest down were: 8,962 French; 3,113 Polish; 300 Italians; 2,341 North Americans; 2,217 Germans; 2,095 Balkan; 1,853 British; 1,722 Belgians; 1,066 Czechs. Michel Lefébvre and Rémi Skoutlesky, *Les Brigades Internationales. Images Retrouvées* (Paris, France: Seuil, 2003), 16.

8. Oscar Telge, "Prólogo," in *Nuestra Lucha Contra La Muerte. El Trabajo del Servicio Sanitario Internacional*, ed. Jirku Gusti (nickname Augusta Franciska Stridsberg; no editorial data, 1937), 8.

9. Report on the Medical Service of International Brigades dated in Barcelona on 26 November 1937, Archivo del Servicio Histórico Militar, Madrid, Spain, (file 1265, Folder 11). Quoted by Jesús Bescos Torres, "Las enfermeras en la Guerra de España (1936–1939)," *Revista de Historia Militar* 26 (1992): 97–143.

10. Gloria Gallego-Caminero et al., "La Historiografía Sobre Las Enfermeras en Las Brigadas Internacionales (1936–1939). Una Revisión Sistemática." Poster presented at ICN Conference and CNR, La Valletta, Malta, May 2011; Gloria Gallego-Caminero et al., "75 Years Later. International Solidarity: Nurses of the International Brigades in The Spanish Civil War (1936–1939)." (Oral presentation, Internacional Nursing History Conference, Kolding, Denmark, August 12, 2012; Gloria Gallego-Caminero, "Al Servicio de las Ideas. Religiosas y militantes," in *Al servicio de las ideas. La Enfermería en los Procesos Populares de Liberación en Iberoamérica*, ed. Beatriz Morrone (Mar del Plata, Argentina: Ediciones Suárez, 2013), 199–234; Sioban Nelson and Gloria Gallego-Caminero, "Beyond the Fiction and Myths: Revisiting the Question of Nurses and Nursing in the International Brigades of the Spanish Civil War (1936–1939)." (Oral presentationat 32nd Annual AAHN Nursing & Health Care History Conference, Dublin, Ireland, September 17–20, 2015); Gloria Gallego-Caminero, Sioban Nelson, and Paola Galbany-Estragues, "Enfermeras internacionales en la Guerra Civil española (1936–1939)," in *Libro del XIV Congreso Nacional y IX Internacional de Historia de la Enfermería. Un siglo cuidando a la sociedad. Centenario del reconocimiento oficial de la Enfermería en España*, eds. M. L. Fernández, A. C. García Martínez, and M. J. García Martínez (Santander, Spain: Colegio de Enfermería de Cantabria, Universidad de Cantabria, 2015), 347–52.

11. Mary Birgham de Urquidi, *Misericordia en Madrid* (México: Costa-Amic, 1975); Lini de Vries, *Up from the Cellar. An Autobiography* (Minneapolis, MN: Vanilla

Press, 1976); Judith Keene, *The last Mile to Huesca: An Australian Nurse in the Spanish Civil War* (Kensington, Australia: South Wales University Press, 1988), Published in Spanish: Judith Keene and Victor Pardo Lancina, eds, *Agnes Hodson, A una Milla de Huesca. Diario de una enfermera australiana en la Guerra Civil Española* (Zaragoza, Spain: Universidad de Zaragoza, 2005); Penelope Fyvel, *English Penny* (Devon: Arthur H. Stockwell Ltd., 1992); Angela Jackson, *For Us It Was Heaven,* Published in Spanish: Angela Jackson, *Para nosotros era el cielo. Pasión dolor y fortaleza de Patience Darton: de la guerra civil española a la China de Mao* (Barcelona, Spain: Ediciones San Juan de Dios Campus Docent, 2012); Mark Derby, *Petals and Bullets Dorothy Morris New Zealand Nurse in the Spanish Civil War* (Brighton, Chicago, Toronto: Susex Academic Press, 2015).

12. Jim Fyrth, *The Signal was Spain. The Spanish Aid Movement in Britain, 1936–39* (London, UK: Lawrence and Wishart, 1986); Frances Patai, "Heroines of the Good Fight. Testimonies of U.S. Volunteer Nurses in the Spanish Civil War, 1936–1939," *Nursing History Review* 3 (1995): 76–104; Nicholas Coni, *Medicine and Warfare. Spain, 1936–1939* (New York: Routledge, 2008), 31–33; Maria del Carmen Pérez-Aguado et al., ""Medicine and Nursing in the Spanish Civil War: Women Who Served in the Health Services of the International Brigades (1936-1939)," *Vesalius: Acta Internationales Historiae Medicinae* (2010): 29–33; Linda Palfreeman, *¡Salud! British Volunteers in the Republican Medical Service during the Spanish Civil War, 1936–1939* (Brighton, UK: Sussex Academic Press, 2012); Angela Jackson, *British Women and the Spanish Civil War* (Abingdon, UK: Routledge, 2002); Walter J. Lear, "American medical support for Spanish Democracy, 1936–1938," in *Comrades in Health: U.S. Health Internationalists, Abroad and at Home*, eds. Anne-Emanuelle Birn and Theodore M. Brown (New Brunswick, NJ: Rutgers University Press, 2013), 65–81; Anne-Emanuelle Birn and Theodore M. Brown, "Across the Generations: Lesson from Health Internationalism," in *Comrades in Health: U.S. Health Internationalists, Abroad and at Home*, eds. Anne-Emanuelle Birn and Theodore M. Brown (New Brunswick, NJ: Rutgers University Press, 2013), 303–18.

13. George Orwell, *Homage to Catalonia* (Middletown, DE: Dogstail Books, 2015), 145.

14. "Annie Murray Obituary," *The Herald Scotland,* 4 December, 1996. www.heraldscotland.com/news/1n.d.052.Annie_Murrie/. The documents have both her English and Scottish (Murrie) name listed. Accessed 11 June, 2019.

15. Jackson, *For Us It Was Heaven*, 27. This quote has been much cited. Originally this very critical assessment of the religious nursing sisters came from Roser Valls, ed., *Infermeres catalanes a la Guerra Civil espanyola* (Barcelona, Spain: Edicions Universistat de Barcelona, 2008), 23. The Valls quote presents the testimony of a Communist Party nurse who (perhaps unsurprisingly) paints an unflattering picture of religious nurses.This same quote turns up in Palfreeman's book. Linda Palfreeman, *Aristocrats, Adventurers and Ambulances. British Medical Units in the Spanish Civil War* (Brighton, Chicago, Toronto: Sussex Academic Press, 2015).

16. Ruth Wilson, Radio Speech from Madrid on January 10, 1938 (Marx Memorial Library Box D-2: A / 1). Identifying the IB nurses is challenging. For instance Ruth Epstein appears in the sources as a Canadian and an American, as Jewish and as married to a Jewish man, under the names of Esther and Ruth, Wilson and Epstein. According to Francisco Guerra she was Esther WILSON (1906–1996), a single woman born in Toronto, Canada. She was a registered nurse who in 1934 married Jake Epstein, who also came to Spain. She arrived May 29, 1937. After joining the IB she was appointed sergeant, head nurse of

the "Centro" hospital in Murcia, from there she went to the "Universidad" hospital and finally to the "Red House" hospital. She was evacuated in April 1938 to the Hospital de Mataró, Barcelona, from there to Vich, Barcelona and repatriated in August in 1938. She died in New York. Francisco Guerra, *La Medicina en el exilio republicano* (Madrid, Spain: Universidad de Alcalá, 2003), 508.

17. Jackson, *For Us It Was Heaven*, 28, 30, 46. Jackson does allow that the Catalan government "Began an Ambitious Project for Training Nurses, the First School Having Opened in Barcelona in 1933," 27.

18. However, Darton is full of admiration for the innovative Catalan surgeons, especially Moises Broggi and Josep Trueta. Jackson, *For Us It Was Heaven*, 53.

19. Fyrth, *The Signal was Spain*, 45.

20. Palfreeman, *Aristocrat Adventurers and Ambulances*, 155.

21. See for background and quality of the work of the nuns in Spain Gloria Gallego-Caminero, "Celebrando un centenario más allá de los mitos," in *Centenario Enfermeria, 17 Diciembre 2015*, ed. Pilar Almansa (Murcia, Spain: Universidad de Murcia, 2015), 11–27.

22. One of the most important medical advances that occurred in the GCE and later had a widespread use in the Second World War was the use of blood transfusion from bottled and refrigerated blood. The world's first preserved blood-transfusion service was created by the health services of the Republican side in Barcelona (August 1936–January 1939) and directed by Federico Duran Jordà who managed to get 28,900 donors and prepare 9,000 liters of blood for donations). He pioneered the development of field transport to the front of refrigerated blood for transfusions. Frederic Duran Jordà, "El Servici de Transfusió de Sang al Front. Organització-utillatge," in *La Medicina Catalana. Portaveu de l'Occitània Mèdica* Llibreria Catalonia, Barcelona (Abril-maig, 1937), 512–16; Frederic Duran Jordà, "The Barcelona Blood-Transfusion Service," *The Lancet* 233, no. 6031 (1939): 773–75.

23. The abandoning of patients by the nuns is something of an overgeneralization. Accounts by Spanish nurses also refer to sisters who stayed in place, wore civilian clothes and risked grave danger to stay working in the hospitals. Anna Ramió and Carme Torres, eds., *Enfermeras de Guerra* (Barcelona, Spain: Ed. San Juan de Dios, 2015), 204; Carles Hervas I. Puyal, "Sanitat a Catalunya Durant la República i la Guerra Civil," (Tesi doctoral diss., Universitat Pompeu Fabra, 2004). http://www.tdx.cat/bitstream/handle/10803/7467/tchp.pdf?sequence=1&isAllowed=y. Accessed 11 June, 2019.

24. The Infectious Hospital of Valencia was installed in the convent of San Cristobal, which was seized from the Canossian Augustinian nuns. It was built at the end of the nineteenth century to accommodate a religious community, not a hospital. When Patience Darton was there it had been transformed into hospital for few months only and while it was likely not a model of neatness and organization, Darton's claims of years of accumulated waste were highly exaggerated. Jackson, *For Us It Was Heaven*, 33. Another hospital mentioned by Darton was the Pasionaria of Valencia at the Salesian College. It was founded by the Communist Party in November 1936. At the beginning of 1937 it was transformed into the Military Hospital Number 2 with 300 beds. Xavier Garcia Ferrandis and A. J. Munayco, "La evolución de la Sanidad Militar en Valencia durante la Guerra Civil Española (1936–1939)," *Sanidad Militar* 67, no. 4 (2011): 383–89. http://scielo.isciii.es/pdf/sm/v67n4/historia_humanidades.pdf. Accessed 11 June, 2019.

25. Manuel Álvarez, *The Tall Soldier, 40 Years Looking for the Man Who Saved My Life* (Toronto, Canada: Virgo Press, 1980), 69.

26. Isabel Anton-Solanas, Ann Wakefield and Christine Hallett, "International Nurses to the Rescue: The Role and Contribution of the Nurses of the International Brigades during the Spanish Civil War," *Japan Journal of Nursing Science* 16, no.2 (2019): 103–114. doi:10.1111/jjns.12218.

27. Ibid.

28. See a discussion of the providing care during the war in Documents Del Memorial Democratic, *LLums Enmig La Barbàrie Memòries Sobre el Salvament de Vides durant la Guerra Civil a Catalunya (Shining Beacons in the Darkness. Memories of Saving of Lives during the Spanish Civil War in Catalonia*; (Barcelona, Spain: Memorial democràtic. Publicacions de la Generalitat de Catalunya, 2013).

29. For a history of the Spanish nursing profession see Carmen Domínguez-Alcón, in *Los Cuidados y la Profesión Enfermera en España* (Barcelona, Spain: Pirámide, 1986); and in English see Anna Ramió Jofre and Carme Torres Penella, "Nurses: Caring in Times of War," in *LLums Enmig la Barbàrie*, 297–99.

30. Domínguez-Alcón, *Los Cuidados y la Profesión Enfermera en España* (Barcelona, Spain: Pirámide, 1986), 308–11.

31. Ibid.

32. Ibid.

33. Rosa Pulido Mendoza, *"La Formación de Las Enfermeras de la Cruz Roja Española: Legado Histórico-filosófico."* Tesi doctoraldiss, Universidad Complutense, Madrid, 2008).

34. Delores Martín Moruno and Javier Ordóñez Rodríguez, "Nursing Vocation as Political participation for Women during the Spanish Civil War," *Journal of War and Cultural Studies* 2, no. 3 (2009): 305–19.

35. Mercedes Milá Molla was a key figure in Spanish nursing of the period. She received a Rockefeller Foundation fellowships in 1931 and 1936, and attended the program conducted at Belford College, University of London for international nursing leaders. During the Civil War she was the only woman member of the Nationalist general headquarters of *Generalisimo*, served as President of the Cruz Roja women and was responsible for the management of the General Inspectorate of the Female Hospital Services. Mercedes Milá Nolla, "La mujer en la Guerra: enfermeras," in *Los médicos y la Medicina en la Guerra Civil Española*, ed. Monografías Beecham (Madrid, Spain: Sanidad Ediciones, 1986), 303–8; Navarro Carballo, "Doña Mercedes Milá Nolla y el Cuerpo de Damas Auxiliares Sanidad Militar. Entrevista del 5 de octubre de 1985," *Sanidad Militar* 43, no. 2 (1987): 332–36; Nicholas Coni, "The Head of all the Nurses," *International Journal of Iberian Studies* 22, no. 1 (2009): 79–84; Josep Bernabeu Mestre, Perez Gascón, and Ma. Encarnoción, *Historia de la Enfermería de Salud Pública* (Publiccaiones de la Universidad de Alicante, Alicante, 1999); Carmen Torres Penella et al., "Relats. Las Enfermeras catalanas en la Guerra Civil española," *Temperamentum* 6 (2007), http://www.index-f.com/temperamentum/tn6/t2707.php. Accessed 11 June, 2019.

36. Carmen Domínguez-Alcón, *Los Cuidados y la Profesión Enfermera en España* (Barcelona, Spain: Pirámide, 1986), 120–21; Carmen Domínguez-Alcón, *La infermeria a Catalunya* (Barcelona, Spain: Editorial Rol, 1986), 26.

37. Bernabeu and Gascón, *Historia de la Enfermería de Salud Pública*; Cronos, "Cuadernos valencianos de historia de la medicina y de la ciencia," *ISSN 1139-711X* 3, no. 1 (2000): 219–21. For a discussion of public health and Settlement nursing in the

United States see Patricia D'Antonio, *American Nursing, The History of Knowledge, Authority, and the Meaning of Work* (Baltimore, MD: Johns Hopkins Press, 2010), 64–72.

38. José Ramón Navarro Carballo, "Creación y desarrollo del Cuerpo de Damas de Sanidad Militar," *Medicina Militar* 43, no. 1987, 320–31.

39. Gaston Leval, *Le Espagne Libertaire 1936–1939: L'ouvre Constructive de la Revolutión Espagnole* (Paris, France: Editions du Cercle, 1971); Cited by Thomas, *The SCW*, 536.

40. Martín Maruno and Ordóñez Rodríguez, "The Nursing Vocation as Political Participation."

41. Hernández Conesa, Juana María, and Gabriel Segura, López, "La formación de las damas enfermeras de la Cruz Roja durante la guerra civil española (1936–1939)," *Index de enfermería* 22, no. 3 (2013): 180–83. For a discussion of the divergent ideologies of the Cruz Roja on the Government and Rebel sides see Maruno and Rodríguez, "The Nursing Vocation as Political Participation."

42. Maruno and Rodríguez, "The Nursing Vocation as Political Participation," 317.

43. Carmen Rivera Villegas, "Otras Miradas Sobre la Guerra Civil Española: Tina Modotti y Elena Garro," *Bulletin of Hispanic Studies* 81, no. 3 (2004): 347–60.

44. Valls, *Infermeres catalanes*, 45.

45. Anna Ramió Jofre et al., *Enfermeras de Guerra* (Barcelona, Spain: San Juan de Dios, Campus Docent, 2015).

46. Documents Del Memorial Democratic, No. 3, *Shining Beacons in the Darkness*.

47. Neither were the international volunteers exempt from such scrutiny, one Australian nurse, Agnes Hodson, who was avowedly apolitical came under strong suspicion from a communist compatriot, Mary Lowson, because she spoke Italian and was well educated. Hodson experienced delays in being deployed to the front. Amirah Inglis, *Australians in the Spanish Civil War* (Sydney, Australia: Allen & Unwin, 1987), 41, 61. Physicians were subject to the same suspicions. Many of them switched sides when they had the chance.

48. Pibernat, "Mis Memorias."

49. For a discussion of public health in Spain see Rafael Huertas, "Política Sanitaria de la Dictadura de Primo de Rivera a la II República," *Revista Española de Salud Pública* 74 (2000), http://scielo.isciii.es/scielo.php?pid=S1135-57272000000600004&script=sci_arttext, accessed 11 June, 2019; Esteban Rodriguez-Ocaña, *Salud Pública en España. Ciencia, profesión y política, siglos XVIII-XX* (Granada, Spain: Universidad de Granada, 2005), 12–80; Roser Valls et al., *Infermeres catalanes a la Guerra Civil española* (Barcelona, Spain: Universitat de Barcelona, 2008), 23; For a discussion of public health nursing initiatives in Spain and the impact of international initiatives on the Spanish context see María Eugenia Galiana-Sánchez, "History of Public Health Nursing in Spain and the International Context," *European Journal for Nursing History and Ethics* 1 (2019): 124–41.

50. The worst of the bombing was by German aircraft which took place on February 3, 1939 attacking unarmed refugees fleeing to France through a narrow area bounded by the sea and the mountains, 83 people died, of whom 49 adults and 25 children could not be identified. Joan Villarroya, "El Bombardeig de Figueras," in *La Guerra Civil a Catalunya 1936–1939*, 62nd ed. eds. Josep Maria Solé i Sabaté and Joan Villarroya (Barcelona, Spain: 2005), 766–69.

51. Roser Valls, "Mas alla de la profesion: Trinidad Gallego Prieto," in *Enfermeras de Guerra*, ed. Ramió and Torres, (Ediciones San JUan de Dios, Campus Docent, Barcelona, 2015) 177–89.

52. Carme Torres and Roser Valls, "Realidad y ficción: Maria Sans Moyà," in *Enfermeras de Guerra*, ed. Ramió and Torres, 118–23.

53. Ibid.

54. For a discussion of nursing as a form of political engagement for women during the Republic and the war see Maruno and Rodríguez, "The Nursing Vocation as Political Participation," 305–19; Pilar Díaz Sánchez, "Las enfermeras de Guerra: otra forma de participación política de las mujeres," *Temperamentum* 2 (2005): 1, http://www.index-f.com/temperamentum/tn2/t0611.php. Accessed 11 June, 2019.

55. Austrian nurse Auguste Guttman had participated in the Great War. She arrived in Spain in August 1937 and remained until the evacuation of Catalonia. She worked at the Hospital of Villanueva de la Jara. Fellow Austrian Anna Peczenik was a nurse at the rearguard hospital in Benicàssim. Both women were murdered by the National Socialists in the concentration camps together with their Spanish Civil War veteran husbands Fritz Guttman and Herman Peczenik. Hans Landauer, *Diccionario de Los Voluntarios Austriacos en la España Republicana 1936–1939* (Madrid, Spain: Asociación de Amigos de las Brigadas Internacionales, 2005).

56. Ibid.

57. Aurora Edenhaffer Documents, International Brigades Archives (IBA 29/D/1) in Marx Memorial Library, London.

58. Guerra, *La Medicina en el exilio republicano*; Encarna Gascón, María Eugenia Galina, and Josep Bernabeu, *El Exilio Científico Republicano* cap. III, ed. Josep L. Barona (Valencia, Spain: Universidad de Valencia, 2010), 99–130; For the situation of exiled midwives see Dolores Rúiz Verdún and Alberto Gomis, "Las Matronas Españolas en El Exilio," *Quipu* 14, no. 2 (2012): 221–38.

59. Pibernat, "Mis Memorias," 63.

60. Valls, "Mas alla de la profesion," 177–89.

61. Torres and Valls, "Realidad y ficción," 123.

62. Margalida Miró et al., "Spanish Nursing under Franco: Reinvention, Modernization and Repression (1956–1976)," *Nursing Inquiry* 19, no. 3 (2012): 270–80.

63. Carmen Torres and Roser Valls, "Infermeria durant la Guerra Civil," in *Infermeres Catalanes*, ed. Valls et al. (1975), 27. The Government of the *Generalitat* decreed on 12 June 1937 that people with nursing titles acquired through unofficial channels should pass an additional examination in order to receive a certificate of official competition that would replace all other qualifications (diplomas, titles, etc.) obtained. The Social Service was mandatory for all women between 17 and 35 years, for a minimum of 6 months and was organized and tutored by the *Sección Femenina de Falange* (Female Section of Falange Party, the party that supported the Nationalists). It was a prerequisite for all women who wished to obtain a degree to pursue a career, work in public and private companies, public jobs or get driving license. Nurses were generally exempt from Social Service. It was abolished at the death of Franco in 1975.

64. Pilar Almansa Martínez, "La formación enfermera desde la Sección Femenina," *Enfermería Global* 7 (2005): 1–11 www.um.es/ojs/index.php/eglobal/article/viewFile/484/468. Accessed 11 June, 2019 ; Anna Ramió Jofre and Carme Torres Penella, "Nurses: Caring in Times of War," in *Documents Del Memorial*

Democratic Shining Beacons in the Darkness, 296–310; Carles Hervas I. Puyal, *Catalonia's Doctors and the Spanish Civil War (1936–39)*, *Ibid*. Both texts includes testimonies from veteran Catalan nurses and doctors from a variety of backgrounds and levels of training.

65. Dr. JoséSiles, Prologo, in Beatriz Morrone (compiladora) "Al Servicio de las ideas," in *La Enfermería en los Procesos Populares de Liberación en Iberoamérica*, 2nd ed. (Argentina: Ediciones Suárez, 2013), 9.

66. Miró et al., "Spanish Nursing under Franco," 270–80.

67. Ibid.

68. Ibid.

69. Pibernat, "Mis Memorias," 37–63.

Disclosure. The authors have no relevant financial interest or affiliations with any commercial interests related to the subjects discussed within this article.

Sioban Nelson, RN, PhD, FAAN, FCAHS
Professor
Lawrence S. Bloomberg Faculty of Nursing
University of Toronto
155 College Street
Toronto, ON
M5T 1P8, Canada

Paola Galbany-Estragués, PhD
Research Group on Methodology, Methods, Models and Outcomes of Health and Social Sciences (M3O)
Faculty of Health Science and Welfare
Centre for Health and Social Care Research
University of Vic-Central University of Catalonia
C. Sagrada Família, 7, 08500 Vic, Spain

Gloria Gallego-Caminero, RN, BA, PhD
Honorary Collaborating Professor
Department of Nursing and Physiotherapy
University of Balearic Island
Ctra de Valldemosa Km 7,5 Palma, Spain

The Norwegian Mobile Army Surgical Hospital in the Korean War (1951–1954): Military Hospital or Humanitarian "Sanctuary?"

Jan-Thore Lockertsen
UiT –The Arctic University of Norway

Åshild Fause
UiT –The Arctic University of Norway

Christine E. Hallett
The University of Huddersfield

Abstract. During the Korean War (1950–1953) the Norwegian government sent a mobile army surgical hospital (MASH) to support the efforts of the United Nations (UN) Army. From the first, its status was ambiguous. The US-led military medical services believed that the "Norwegian Mobile Army Surgical Hospital" (NORMASH) was no different from any other MASH; but both its originators and its staff regarded it as a vehicle for humanitarian aid. Members of the hospital soon recognized that their status in the war zone was primarily that of a military field hospital. Yet they insisted on providing essential medical care to the local civilian population as well as trauma care to UN soldiers and prisoners of war. The ambiguities that arose from the dual mission of NORMASH are explored in this article, which pays particular attention to the experiences of nurses, as expressed in three types of source: their contemporary letters to their Matron-in-Chief; a report written by one nurse shortly after the war; and a series of oral history interviews conducted approximately 60 years later. The article concludes that the nurses of NOR-MASH experienced no real role-conflict. They viewed it as natural that they should offer their services to both military and civilian casualties according to need, and they experienced a sense of satisfaction from their work with both types of patient. Ultimately, the experience of Norwegian nurses in Korea

Nursing History Review 28 (2020): 93–126. A Publication of the American Association for the History of Nursing. Copyright © 2020 Springer Publishing Company.
http://dx.doi.org/10.1891/1062-8061.28.93

illustrates the powerful sense of personal agency that could be experienced by nurses in forward field hospitals, where political decision-making did not impinge too forcefully on their clinical and ethical judgment as clinicians.

The Korean War and the Norwegian Mobile Army Surgical Hospital

During The Korean War (1950–1953), Norwegian medical and nursing personnel operated a Norwegian Mobile Army Surgical Hospital (NORMASH) close to the front lines of conflict. The purpose of this article is to explore the ambiguities inherent in NORMASH. It addresses the question: how and why did Norway's small mobile field hospital provide both military surgical expertise and humanitarian aid during the Korean War? The main focus of our study was on the work of nurses, and we were particularly interested in exploring their influence in molding the hospital's humanitarian emphasis. The purpose of this article is to offer insights into the ways in which the Norwegian nurses' sense of personal agency influenced the dual mission of NORMASH. Hence, it also addresses a number of supplemental questions: How and why did Norwegian nurses come to serve in a war zone far from their homeland? How did they cope with the challenges they met in Korea? And, how did their sense of themselves, as professional nurses, influence the ways in which they responded to working within the highly militaristic environment of a mobile army surgical hospital (MASH)?

The Korean War began on 25 June 1950, when North Korea attacked South Korea by crossing the 38th parallel, practically overrunning its neighboring country in a swift and decisive operation.[1] In a counter strike, a US-led United Nations (UN) Army drove the North Korean People's Army almost to the border of China. Then, in yet another wave of aggression, China entered the war and forced the UN army to withdraw to the 38th parallel. Here, the war entered a new phase as a gruelling trench war.[2] It was during this phase that NORMASH was operative—an active unit from July 1951 until 1 year after the armistice—eventually closing in October 1954. It was first located near Uijongbu in a beautiful orchard, a place so striking that the hospital came to be known as "The Orchard." Then, in September 1951, NORMASH moved to Tongduchon closer to the battle zone. On 24 June 1952, the hospital moved for the last time, to a location just over 4 kilometers to the north where it could be better defended.[3]

The hospital's Norwegian founders originally intended it to be a civilian hospital. It then developed into a military unit, before it entered a long phase during which it exhibited characteristics of both a military hospital and a center for humanitarian aid. It was the last mobile hospital to enter the Korean War; it was also the last such hospital to leave the former battlefields. Toward the end of its time, it served little military purpose, but functioned mainly as a civilian hospital for Koreans.

NORMASH developed in several phases, from a Red Cross Hospital and center for humanitarian aid, to a military hospital, and then to a "hybrid hospital" where both soldiers and civilians were treated. These phases went beyond the inevitable evolution of a unit in response to the changing conditions of war. They appear to have been driven—at least in part —by the powerful sense of agency which enabled nurses to fulfil what they saw as a humanitarian mission. The present study of NORMASH is the first scholarly work to examine nurses' practices at NORMASH during the Korean War.

Before the Second World War, Norway had been a neutral country, but, following that war, it abandoned its neutrality—a response that may have been evoked by its experience of occupation by Nazi Germany. The Norwegian government interpreted its involvement in the Korean War not as a belligerent move, but, rather, as an attempt to bring peace to a troubled region.[4] In the event, this was the first war on foreign soil in which Norway participated. Some Norwegian sources discuss the Korean War as a part of the Cold War and view it as the spark that hastened the development the Norwegian armed forces.[5] Memoirs and diaries adopt a more personal tone. Most were written by soldiers or clergymen, and tell intimate stories: the daily life of a soldier, the workings of a scout troop; the establishment of a newspaper. The intention of this article is to add to this body of knowledge by offering observations on the work of a hitherto neglected group: nurses.[6] Memoirs, for all their eclectic and slightly random content can offer insights into the ways in which people gave meaning to their work. They were among a range of sources mobilized by this study, to give a broad insight into the operation of NORMASH. Alongside them, we placed the official documents, originally lodged in the archive of the Norwegian Armed Forces Medical Services Collection. Many of these records have been handed over to Riksarkivet, the National Archives of Norway, and can be found in Box RAFA, File 3422. The collection includes official reports produced during the war, and a variety of private letters written by nurses to their Matron-in-Chief. These letters give insight into how nurses perceived their daily life during their 6-month assignments in Korea, and enable an understanding of some of the ways in which they gave meaning to their work as both expert practice and humanitarian mission. Some of the letters were written during the nurses' stay in Korea, others shortly after their return to Norway.[7]

Oral history interviewing was a key component of the study, and we were mindful of the intended purposes of the methodology—a rigorous discipline which developed in the late twentieth century.[8] This is the first major study of the experiences, work, and perspectives of nurses at the Korean NOR-MASH. Very few histories have focussed on the agency of women in war zones or within humanitarian relief organizations. One notable exception is Susan Armstrong-Reid and David Murray's *Armies of Peace*, which recounts the memories of so-called "UNRRAIDS," and illustrates the ways in which they believed they were able to make a positive difference to the provision of aid, in spite of bureaucratic in-fighting at the UN Relief and Rehabilitation Administration.[9] Another is Yihong Pan's 2014 paper, "Never a Man's War," which focuses on the involvement of the women soldiers of the New Fourth Army in the Chinese War of Resistance against Japan (1937–1945). Pan's paper explores the ways in which women's own writings could "human-ize" female war-participants. Her sources enabled her to gain a sense of "their daily life and work from gendered perspectives, in contrast to the Maoist stereotyped super heroine images of Communist women." Her work stresses the importance of studying women's own writings in order to capture their "own agency" adding that her reading of their personal writings convinced her that "to [these women], the war was never a man's cause."[10] Pan's re-ordering of historical categories is quite radical, and her perspective differs from ours in significant ways. Her emphasis on the link between personal writings and historical understandings of personal agency has, nevertheless, influenced our own work. The letters and accounts of the nurses who served at NORMASH, lodged in the Norwegian State Archives alongside the oral history interviews, captured these women's sense of their own personal agency, and opened-up new ways of interpreting events at NORMASH that could emphasize, for the first time, the perspectives of nurses.[11]

The History of the "Front-Line" Hospital and the Formation of NORMASH

The twentieth century saw a tremendous development in warfare from the engagement of standing armies in clearly defined and contained conflicts to the involvement of mass civilian armies fighting over vast swathes of terri-tory. The engagement of civilian volunteer armies focused the attention of whole populations on the survival and welfare of troops and encouraged sup-port for army medical services. The rapid transportation of wounded service-men from battlefields to hospitals was soon recognized as being crucial to their survival. Full scale conflicts, such as the so-called "Great War" from 1914 to 1918, brought recognition of the need to bring medical aid closer to the battle zone. This led to the development of mobile hospitals that could be deployed close to the frontline. The British Royal Army Medical Corps introduced casualty clearing hospitals that were later to be called casualty clearing stations (CCSs). These small field hospitals, located between field ambulances and stationary hospitals, were designed to offer first-line treatment—in particular to remove debris from wounds, and perform life-saving surgical procedures such as amputations—and they could host several hundred casualties.[12]

During the First World War the French Service de Santé des Armées, experimented with surgical units more mobile than CCSs. Autochirs— Ambulances Chirurgical Automobile—provided forward surgery even closer to the battlefield. The French idea was adopted by the US Army during the later years of the war.[13] The Second World War was more mobile than the First, and created a need for even more mobile units, known as auxiliary surgery groups (ASGs), which were associated with further reductions in mortality rates.[14] MASHs grew out of these developments; they were 60-bed hospitals which were designed to be highly mobile and were located 6–15 miles from the front between battalion aid stations and evacuation hospitals.[15] The Korean War is closely associated with their use.[16]

The contributions of military nurses in small field hospitals during the Korean War have received very little scholarly attention. The war has been called "the Forgotten War," and Quincealea Brunk argues that it was an unpopular service for Americans.[17] Mary Sarnecky quotes First Lieutenant Mary C. Quinn expressing the same view. Quinn had served with the US 8055 MASH and had arrived at the front at about the same time as NORMASH became operational. She experienced a barrier in communication about the war with people in the United States, finding that the Korean War was not a war people wanted to hear about.[18]

Earlier work on nurses' perspectives has been largely descriptive, often bordering on the celebratory. Two short articles in *The American Journal of Nursing*, "With the Army Nurse Corps in Korea," and "With the First MASH," give insights into both the conditions in Korea and the nature of peri-operative nursing.[19] One interesting autobiography of "The Forgotten War" is a memoir by British nurse, Jill McNair. Her experience as a nurse in the Korean War relates to the British Commonwealth General Hospital in Kure, Japan, and the British Commonwealth Zone Medical Unit in Seoul, Korea; she never served in a MASH.[20] Military historian, Eric Taylor focuses on nursing at an evacuation hospital in Pusan and on a hospital ship, rather than in a MASH close to the battlefield.[21] His focus is also on British nurses and his approach is celebratory rather than analytical, as is that of Frances Omori, who offers a narrative of navy nurses and hospital ships.[22] A small number of articles have focussed on clinical developments, identifying medical advances, such as helicopter evacuation of causalities and technical improvements in blood bank services, as outcomes of the conflict.[23]

The Norwegian Red Cross was founded in 1865; its purpose was voluntary medical aid in war and support to the Army's Medical Services.[24] However, it had little involvement in international medical aid in war until 1912.[25] From then until 1940 the Norwegian Red Cross endowed ambulances staffed with trained nurses in four different military conflicts: The First Balkan War (1912–1913); The Finnish Civil War (27 January–15 May 1918); the Second Italo-Ethiopian War (1935–1936); and The Winter War between Soviet Union and Finland (30 November 1939–13 March 1940).[26]

The Norwegian field hospital in Korea was, initially, a Red Cross hospital administered by the Ministry of Foreign Affairs. Official histories of both the Norwegian Red Cross and the Armed Forces Medical Services mention the hospital, which was transformed into a military hospital under the control of the Ministry of Defence.[27] Kjetil Skorand mentions NORMASH, but does not consider the role of nurses or nursing.[28] Kaare Gulbransen a veteran from the ambulance in Ethiopia (1935–1936), the Ambulance in Finland (1939–1940), and The Norwegian Field Hospital in Korea (Contingent One, 1951), commented that no histories had explored the meaning of "surgeons' and nurses' hard work day and night, under conditions that were both difficult, unfamiliar and primitive."[29]

The birth of NORMASH was turbulent. From 1947 onward tensions between the United States, the Soviet Union, and their respective allies increased, and Europe became divided by what has been termed an "Iron Curtain" separating east and west blocks from 1948 to about 1990. In 1949, Norway joined the defensive alliance, known as the North Atlantic Treaty Organization (NATO). It was, at that time, the only NATO country that shared a border with the Soviet Union. In 1950, with the outbreak of the Korean War, the so-called Cold War was said to have become "hot."[30] Norway was one of the countries that had endorsed the UN' decision to oppose any aggression from North Korea against South Korea. The Secretary-General of the UN, Trygve Lie—himself a Norwegian citizen—had referred to this as a "constabulary action."[31] Norway was asked to participate in what was, without doubt, a military operation, but, in the early 1950s, the Norwegian armed forces were still under reconstruction after almost 5 years of occupation (June 10, 1940 to May 8, 1945) during the Second World War. Hence, although there was nothing that indicated any threats in Northern Europe, The Norwegian government believed that its armed forces were needed at home and it refused to participate in the military operation, instead offering to support the Korean people with a refugee camp and a hospital.[32] Pressure was exerted on the Norwegian government by both the UN and the United States, to participate with armed forces, and, as a compromise, it eventually agreed to send a field hospital.[33] The Ministry of Foreign Affairs gave the task of planning and staffing that hospital to the Norwegian Red Cross—Norges Røde Kors.[34]

The Red Cross had two alternative plans for the organization of the field hospital. The first option was a MASH equipped like a US MASH and staffed with military personnel. The other was a Red Cross hospital staffed with civilian medical personnel serving alongside personnel with auxiliary functions and official status within the Red Cross. The Surgeon General of the Norwegian Armed Forces Medical Services was in favor of the first plan, but the Norwegian Ministry of Defence did not give permission to operate a military hospital in Korea.[35] The Norwegian field hospital was therefore designated as a civil field hospital which would offer treatment and care to combatant servicemen and would serve alongside US MASHs at the front.

The United States was the executive agent for the UN's operation in Korea, and the Norwegian field hospital was tactically placed to support the Eighth US Army in Korea (EUSAK). An agreement between Norway and the United States regulated all practical aspects of the hospital's daily operation. All supplies were to be provided by the United States.[36] In practice this meant that almost everything except personal items were of US origin. The agreement also specified that NORMASH personnel would follow orders handed down by the commanding general of the Armed Forces of the Member States of the UN in Korea.[37]

This civil Red Cross hospital was operative from July 1951, but only attained the title "The Norwegian Mobile Army Surgical Hospital (NORMASH)" in October 1951. Its main purpose was to serve combatant forces —mainly the Commonwealth Division and the First US Cavalry Division— close to the 38th Parallel. NORMASH served on equal terms with the other MASHs. During their time in Korea US MASHs increased in size from 60-bed hospitals to 200-bed hospitals. In 1951, questions were raised about whether NORMASH, with only 60 beds, was big enough to make a significant contribution.[38] A Norwegian report from November 17, 1951, responded to the challenge by stating that the question of the number of beds at NORMASH was immaterial. The Norwegian detachment served a division like the others and had to take the patients that came in during the rushes; hence, it had to expand as and when necessary.[39]

Heavy fighting, especially in 1951, created a large number of battle casualities. The Norwegian field hospital was much needed and it was later reported that it "pulled its weight."[40] Figures for the period from the hospital's opening on July 19, 1951 to its closing down in October, 1954, suggest that approximately 90,000 individuals were treated, either as inpatients or through the polyclinic (outpatient clinic). Of these, 14,755 were inpatients—12,201 before the armistice and 2,554 between armistice and closure. This suggests that the polyclinic was highly active. Over the total period, more than 9,600 operations were said to have been performed.[41]

The Nurses of NORMASH

Norway has never had a professional army nursing corps. Nurse education in Norway was conducted in public hospitals and in the private schools of charitable organizations. Government grants helped to support both types of schools, and, in return, both were obliged to provide educated nurses for duty during catastrophes and in time of war. Yet, these nurses did not receive any military training.[42] Military field hospitals meant for use in war or during catastrophes were intended to be staffed with personnel mobilized from civil hospitals.[43] During inauguration into Red Cross service, nurses were given a military "dog tag" together with the Red Cross emblem to use if mobilized for service during war.[44]

In 1946, the Norwegian Storting (Norway's parliament) legislated to end all military training for women. This was not reversed until 1953, when women were allowed to attend army schools and courses on a voluntary basis. Nevertheless, there was demand for nursing service in the armed forces built on the engagement of civilian nurses.[45] Between 1947 and 1953, Norway provided approximately 4,000 soldiers to the British Army of the Rhine—the army of occupation in Germany. Each contingent served for 6 months as part of "national service." In every contingent there were 13 nurses: 12 "ward nurses" and 1 "head nurse." In total, 118 nurses served in Germany; others served with the standing army at home.[46]

Many of these experienced nurses went on to serve at NORMASH. Due to their experiences of the occupation, Norwegians in general felt that Norway had a moral obligation to participate in the UN operation to stop aggression from North Korea against South Korea. In addition, Norway was the homeland of UN's first Secretary-General, Trygve Lie. The fact that Norway had been occupied by Nazi Germany has been seen as significant in motivating the Norwegian nurses to volunteer for service in Korea.[47] Most were recruited from civil hospitals. Apart from those who served during The Second World War, none had combat experience.[48] Their prior experience fuelled their motivation: the desire to offer humanitarian aid grew out of experiences of observing the suffering of compatriots.

The personnel at NORMASH changed every 6 months. Seven contingents served; in total there were 111 nurses, 22 deacons, 80 surgeons, 5 dentists, 6 pharmacists, 98 officers/NCOs, and 294 privates.[49] Many privates and some of the officers served in two contingents. Only one of the nurses, Petra Drabløs, served with two contingents. Nurses were unable to get absence of leave for more than 6 months from their work in Norway; some also had family obligations at home.[50] Furthermore, Ruth Andresen, the matron-in-chief of the army wanted as many nurses as possible to gain experience with a field hospital in case the cold war should lead to a more local conflict. She would not recommend that any individual nurse serve for more than 6 months.[51]

Nursing service at NORMASH was demanding. Clinical staff in US MASHs realized that critically wounded patients, who in earlier wars would have been dead upon arrival, were now being admitted to hospitals because of rapid evacuation via helicopters.[52] Nurses at NORMASH soon began to describe similar experiences. For this reason, Andresen favoured nurses with good general practice experience and, ideally, at least 4 years' experience as a theater nurse. Not only did the nurses have to have clinical experience and skills; they also needed to be in good health and be able to sleep in a tent for 6 months. Hence, Andresen and her medical colleagues decided that they should not be more than 40 years old.[53]

The nurses of NORMASH had not been trained to function as part of a military organization.[54] Neither had they any training in war surgery.[55] Yet NORMASH was a hospital in the midst of a war and nurses had to deal with war trauma, as well as accidents and internal medicine. The hospital was not able to treat eye and head injuries. Patients with such injuries were evacuated immediately to the rear. Bulletproof vests made of nylon gave protection for the upper body. Extremity injuries therefore accounted for 70% of the injuries according to Norwegian figures.[56] US sources have claimed that the role of nurses in trauma care developed during the Korean War.[57] US Army nurses were said to have functioned on a much higher level than in a civilian setting; hence, for this reason, Brunk has claimed, war is a catalyst for change in nursing.[58] The lack of trained theater nurses in the US Army led to formal courses in operating room techniques. During the war either a trained nurse or a technician could assist the surgeon during operations at US MASHs.[59]

Norway had not allowed men to train as nurses prior to 1948. It did, however, permit them to undergo a partial training and qualify as so-called "deacons." There were a few exceptions who received full nurse-training. Among these was, Peder Klingsheim, one of the participants interviewed for this study. He received the rank of master sergeant.[60] Some deacons felt that it was unfair that they were not commissioned as officers. But the US Army did not give rank as commissioned officers to male nurses. In a letter from the matron-in-chief, Ruth Andresen, the deacon's work was discussed. None of the deacons were specialist nurses, and Andresen mentioned that the chief surgeon (Arne Hvoslef) for one contingent of NORMASH had said that deacons could not work as theater nurses.[61] Most of them did not have an education that could justify commission as officers.

For NORMASH it seems that the necessity of using fully educated nurses during rushes became clearer as the complexity of the work increased. When a grenade exploded many soldiers threw themselves to the ground. Even though their armored vests protected their upper bodies, shrapnel caused many severe buttock wounds. Pre-operative work was intricate requiring that patients be stabilized prior to surgery. Blood transfusion was required for many patients. "I was the only trained nurse on duty and had to do all the surveillance myself," said Klingsheim.[62] Because of the incidence of adverse reactions, the administration of blood transfusions was work that could be performed only by trained nurses. With regard to the theater nurses, when the first change of contingent came after the home administration of the hospital was transferred from the Red Cross to the army, the staffing was changed and the staffing plan reduced the number of nurses. This worried Arne Hvoslef, the commanding chief of NORMASH, who wrote:

> During the last rush we operated at four tables almost the day around for weeks, and it went well; but you know, the boys (surgeons) were exhausted. And here is another thing: I think the workload was larger for the sisters (theatre nurses). We are using one for anesthesia and one for sterile assistance at each operating table. Then there is no one left for rotation, but they manage because they know that rushes do not last forever.[63]

The nurses in the operating theater had all received specialist training in theater work in Norway. They could not be replaced. They were needed for the most severely wounded. Deacons could, in case of emergency, replace ward nurses, but specialist nurses could not be replaced. Hvoslef reported that the number of trained theater nurses could not be reduced if the MASH were to function as intended.[64] His report gave rise to much discussion in Norway, concerning the need to economize versus the need for properly educated and trained nurses in a war. The Surgeon General of the Armed Forces Medical Services wrote to the Ministry of Defense and expressed his concerns with regard to the question about nurses. NORMASH was in a different situation from US MASHs. Each MASH had a responsibility for casualties in their respective areas of the front. US MASHs could use reserves and depend on a rotation of personnel. NORMASH had no such opportunity. There were no Norwegian reserves in Korea or Japan. The only available staff were those already at the hospital. Most deacons were not fully-trained nurses and could not take over a nurse's work. The number of theater nurses could therefore not be reduced.[65]

Andresen, raised the same problem with the chief of staff. With only eight operating theater nurses in each contingent and a head nurse helping with anesthesia in emergency cases, there was no way the number of theater nurses could be reduced. In fact, she argued for an increase the number of theater nurses. The Brigade in Germany during the late 1940s had had 10 positions for nurses, but they had engaged more in order to enable a rotation of staff.[66] And the Brigade in Germany had not been at war.

The response to the Matron-in-Chief's and the Surgeon General's concern was to grant permission to increase staffing with one surgeon and two nurses if found necessary for daily operations at NORMASH.[67] Another question that was raised by the Matron-in-Chief concerned the injustice of the fact that deacon students—who had not completed their education—were better paid than fully educated nurses. Norway had not allowed nurse education for men prior to 1948. With an education of 3 years (and 2 years of training after that to become a theater nurse), no male nurse could fill a position as theater nurse at NORMASH. Nevertheless, deacons did a valuable job in many places, and some of them had experience from work in Korea or China as missionaries. One reason for using deacons was a wish to have male nurses in the combat zone.[68] The medical officers at NORMASH concluded that nurses could not be substituted with groups with less education.

There were always tasks to do in the hospital that could be handled by personnel without training. A nurse's work went beyond direct patient-care; there was also preparation. Gowning, linen, and instruments are washed, sterilized and stored for use. Gloves were not single-use; they had to be maintained and mended. Such tasks took a lot of time, so even when it was quiet on the front, the hospital worked. It was by performing these routine tasks at quiet times that it could function during rushes. Many of NORMASH's other personnel came after they had finished their daily tasks as drivers or guard soldiers to help with this important work.[69]

Coping with patients' emotional trauma was also an important aspect of nursing care. Hartvigsen commented: "We know so well the feeling, from our daily life and ourselves, the anxiety for illness and pain, for hospital and operation. We saw the same thing here."[70] Soldiers' thoughts about the future and the uncertainty of the outcome of an operation were well understood by theater nurses from their work in civilian hospitals.

Civilian Nurses in a Military Hospital

The nurses at NORMASH were female civilians in a male military culture and were not trained as army nurses. The desire to offer active war-service was not their primary motivation. The Korean War was the first time Norway had participated in such a campaign. All specialist nurses and ward nurses at NORMASH were women, apart from a small number of fully-trained male deacons. NORMASH had started-out as a civil Red Cross hospital and then been transformed into a military hospital. The nurses did not only lack military training; they also lacked experience in war surgery.

In Korea, all nurses had received US Army uniform, and were commissioned as officers in the US Army. The Commanding Chief of the first contingent of NORMASH, Herman Ramstad, was uncomfortable with the arrangement of being a civil hospital, with staff armed and ranked as officers in the US Army. In a report to his superiors in Norway he stated that the hospital had bought carbines and guns, but that it might "be best not to mention that at home." He also wrote that his superiors should consider raising the question of whether NORMASH should be a military hospital, with staff commissioned as officers, formally with the Ministry of Defence.[71] When the Norwegian government became aware, in October 1951, that it had a unit in Korea that in fact operated as a military unit, it insisted that Norwegian nurses and surgeons must be temporarily commissioned officers in the Norwegian Army.[72] However, it did not legislate to enable personnel to wear Norwegian officer's insignia. Throughout the war, the staff of NORMASH continued to wear US officers' insignia.

In retrospect it seems controversial that a Red Cross hospital was transformed into a military hospital; but it may not have been so for the medical personnel. Neither the Red Cross nor the armed forces in Norway believed that an ostensibly civilian hospital could function in the war zone in Korea. Military status was seen as necessary. Early in 1951, the Norwegian Red Cross had a welfare team in Korea—one of several from the League of Red Cross Societies. This team had a similar experience to the staff of NORMASH. Welfare teams were all a part of the United Nations Civil Assistance Command Korea (UNCACK), but the Norwegian team was under the command of EUSAK. All welfare teams had to wear the US Army's battledress without any Red Cross or national emblems. Although the Red Cross protested and demanded to operate as independent welfare teams and not under US military command, their request was denied. The Norwegian team decided to adopt a pragmatic line. Questions about emblems were a question for their organizations. They wore the US Army battledress and carried a card with their rank, stating that this was "Valid only if captured by the enemy."[73] The Norwegian surgeon Carl Semb had in the planning process of NORMASH, held the rank of temporary major general. All negotiations were with military personnel, and officer status was necessary in order that these could take place on equal terms. The Norwegian Red Cross seemed well aware that a hospital would not be able to function at the front without military status.

The Red Cross was founded with the purpose of giving medical aid to sick and wounded soldiers in time of war. Red Cross nurses were all familiar with this ideal. Previous ambulances—apart from "the Balkan Ambulance"—had all operated with military equipment but without ensigns and emblems from the armed forces. It was only afterwards remarked that they were not fully neutral: they always had clear sympathy for one of the sides in the conflicts in which they operated.[74]

Yet nurses resisted militarization in many ways. They had their own hierarchy. In hospitals "Matron-in-Chief" was the highest position among nurses. But the Norwegian nursing profession was also a sisterhood formed through education, work and, a non-militaristic moral discipline. Nurses' letters to their Matron-in-Chief were addressed to "Dear Sister Ruth," and did not use Ruth Andresen's military rank. The rank system in the army was not natural for them. Still, the Norwegian nurses acknowledged its importance when nursing combatant personnel, and adjusted to the military system.

Since the nurses lived in a male society, officer status permitted them to associate with both officers and privates politely and as comrades. Combatants were pleasantly surprised to encounter female nurses in the war zone. A British soldier who had been at NORMASH "was adamant that he had seen female nurses at NORMASH, although he also stated that he could have been hallucinating."[75] Soldiers travelled to the unit's Officers Club and Sergeants Club in the hope of meeting its female staff:

> The fact that NORMASH housed about two dozen beautiful, blonde Norwegian nurses was undoubtedly an added attraction. These were almost never at the club, however (for obvious reasons), so that particular attraction usually faded after a while.[76]

Women reminded soldiers of home and a different life from the trenches, filth, and fighting, but not all soldiers were courteous. Peder Klingsheim, one of the deacons at NORMASH, describes some US soldiers who showed little respect for women: "They used to grab after them, but I guess they were protected by their ranks as commissioned officers."[77] Romances did occur, but they were few. Theater nurse, Margot Isaksen, met her husband-to-be, a guard soldier, in Korea; but her experience was unusual.[78] Mostly, the nurses were somewhat older than the Norwegian soldiers, and appear to have been viewed as mother figures.[79]

Gerd Semb, a veteran of the Second World War and the occupation force in Germany, served at NORMASH as a captain. She recounted a story about how she had been outside the camp, hitchhiking in a military truck. The driver broke the speed limit and was stopped by the military police, but Semb was the one who got reported. "I told him that I had not been driving the car, but he said I was the highest ranked officer and responsible."[80] Semb had not realized that she had authority over the actions of the driver, just because she outranked him. Semb also went to a ceremony in Japan with a private soldier. It was a disappointing experience for them both: where she could go, he could not, and vice versa. She spent the time alone, until she could find a plane back to Korea. The plane was transporting fresh troops on their first mission, and she found a seat between the privates. Then an officer started to admonish the soldiers:

> The young lieutenant gave them a hard speech in foul language. And then he saw that there was a woman among the soldiers. And then he noticed that I was a captain. He was so full of excuses. For the rest of the trip from Japan to Korea I was invited to sit in the cockpit.[81]

Rønnaug Wüller served as head nurse in Korea with the first contingent at NORMASH. She was given the rank of captain and then promoted to major. Afterward she reflected on the fact that without uniform and rank, she would hardly have been able to work as a nurse in a war. Military discipline and respect was gained by rank. There were very few females close to the front-line. For her, the uniform and rank induced the type of respect that was necessary to work as a nurse with male soldiers, something she never had given a thought to before.[82] And rank also provided security if captured by the enemy.

Security was, indeed, an issue. Some questioned whether female nurses should serve in the war zone at all. Major General Carl Semb stated that there had been some very serious and negative experiences for women captured by the enemy, and he did not initially want the hospital too close to the front at the 38th Parallel.[83] The nurses of the first contingent were not ordered to the combat zone in Korea. The matter was discussed with them, and they were given the choice between staying in Pusan or travelling to the combat zone. It was the nurses themselves who volunteered to serve close to the front lines.[84]

From time to time a nurse outranked a surgeon during work in the operating theater. But there was never a question of whether the surgeon was the chief in medical matters. Yet nurses had their seniority too: instructions for private soldiers who were working in the hospital were that they, in every matter that concerned the hospital, were to receive orders from and work under the command of the nurses. This instruction was justified by the superior training of nurses and did not mention that they, as commissioned officers, outranked privates.[85]

NORMASH: A Military or a Humanitarian Endeavor?

The "Orchard" became a legend for NORMASH.[86] After arriving in Pusan, the nurses and other personnel had found themselves in a country riven by war.[87] Yet here, in the midst of the conflict, was an untouched garden —The Orchard —where a haven of hope existed. The sight was described as impressive. After a journey among ruins where only shells of concrete or stone buildings had been left, The Orchard seemed unaffected by the war. It was ripe with apples without scabs or worms, ready to be harvested.[88] Here, NORMASH was established, and officially opened on 19 July 1951.[89] The peaceful surroundings gave opportunities for both sight-seeing and entertaining. Nurse Gerd Semb brought her guitar with her to Korea. She and another nurse, Petra Drabløs, provided entertainment. On one occasion, they were invited to a US MASH. She described their experiences:

> We did not realize that it was a religious gathering, and did not know any religious songs. I said to Petra, let's take "Kom til den hvitmalte kirke" [The Church in the Wildwood]. A popular sing-along and the only song we knew with a religious text. It was not allowed for a nurse to leave the camp without company of a soldier with a gun, but I did it anyway. Once I had a Canadian sergeant drive me to the 38th Parallel. I always felt safe in the Orchard.[90]

The hospital was composed primarily of tents, alongside which were two corrugated iron buildings: a welfare building and a church.[91] This was to be the site for NORMASH for 2 months. It was very quiet along the front during these first months, and very few combatants were wounded in action. Yet there was plenty of work. As Gerd Semb said: "People get sick, also during war."[92] During these early months of the hospital's mission, nurses appear to have felt no sense of conflict: the humanitarian emphasis of their work was to the fore.

The day before the official opening of NORMASH, on July 18, 1951, the first patient was received: a young boy named Pak. The surgeon Bernhard Paus wrote about Pak in his diary:

> July 18, 1951. We received our 1st patient; a 14-year old Korean boy severely burnt a week before. August 27, 1951. Today we brought back the severely burnt boy, Pak. I have been his doctor while he has been here.[93]

This Korean boy was only one of many children who, because of the war, were wounded and in need of specialist healthcare. Pre-war healthcare in South Korea had been limited due to a lack of resources. The war had ruined much of the infrastructure and had left practically nothing.[94] For people living close to the front, NORMASH became a natural place to seek healthcare. The young boy, Pak, was said to have "captured the clinician's hearts." After treatment, he was transported to Seoul, but he wanted to return to NORMASH.[95] Nurse Hetty Henrichsen drove to Seoul to pick him up and bring him back to The Orchard.[96] Many children were helped at NORMASH. Only a few are remembered by name. But Pak's story is not entirely one of success. One day he disappeared; he left without a trace.[97] Bernhard Paus made several attempts to locate him after the war, but was unable to track him down.[98] Not all the children needed surgical help: food, shelter, and a place to sleep were just as likely to be sought at NORMASH.[99]

When the nurses learned about the conditions of the Koreans, they passed on their knowledge to the next contingent. Travelling from Norway to Korea by plane allowed limited weight and for a half-year service everyone needed personal items of different kinds. Along with the official list of what items to bring with them there was, nevertheless, always a request to the new nurses: "The sisters beg the new sisters to bring with them as many clothes as possible for the Koreans, preferably clothes for toddlers."[100]

Caring for children continued after service in Korea. Many nurses continued to collect money and clothes for "our small friends."[101] Also before service in Korea, efforts were made to help children, by providing clothes—sometimes in such amounts that they could not be managed. In a letter to the Matron-in-Chief, a nurse wrote about the trip by plane and seeing Cairo and Bangkok, and then: "My real reason for writing to you is to ask if the children's clothes that I got in Larvik are still in Oslo? They have not been received here [at NORMASH] yet."[102] NORMASH only remained in The Orchard for just over 2 months before it moved closer to the front, to Tongduchon—not as peaceful and romantic as The Orchard, but, strategically, a better location. Yet, it was always The Orchard of which the staff talked.[103]

The Surgeon General of the Norwegian Armed Forces Medical Services had allowed NORMASH to treat civilians who could not reach a Korean hospital. NORMASH often felt a moral obligation not to discharge these patients. The medical needs were of a character that Korean hospitals were not able to offer, ruined as those hospitals were by the war. A report from June 1952 by Colonel Hjort, chief of Hospital Contingent Three, described how surgeons in quiet periods at the front had been sent to Seoul as aid for the Korean Red Cross Hospital. Both the Korean and the Norwegian hospital wanted to continue this cooperation. Surgeons from NORMASH brought their own surgical instruments to Seoul since the Korean hospital lacked such instruments. Colonel Hjort sought advice from the surgeon general on whether this work was to be a priority. The hospital was equipped with surgical instruments for war injuries, but equipment for gynecological intervention, for instance, was not available.[104] The answer from the Surgeon General was that he looked upon humanitarian aid to the civilian population of Korea as very important, and wanted it to be continued. Yet, there must be limits: humanitarian aid had to be limited by NORMASH's primary function as a military surgical field hospital.[105]

Of NORMASH's sixty beds, staff were allowed to use 24 for civilian patients when it was quiet on the front. In reality civilian patients often occupied well over 40% of the beds. At certain times, the average was 35–40 civilian inpatients. Work at the hospital could sometimes be foreseen. If there was rain it would be quiet at NORMASH.[106] If the sound of shooting could be heard in the morning, ambulances would arrive in the afternoon.[107] When battle causalities arrived, civilians could not be evacuated since they had nowhere to go and nothing with which to support themselves. Nurses tried to separate the two groups of patients, sometimes because Korean patients had infectious diseases that were becoming rare in the Western world,[108] but also sometimes for more prosaic and pragmatic reasons: soldiers did not want to lie close to patients who ate garlic,[109] or to share tents with crying babies and old "pappasans" who were, sometimes, spitting on the floor.[110] At the laboratory a nurse remarked that she could hardly find a sample without tuberculosis, and there were times when NORMASH seemed more like a sanatorium than a MASH.[111] In May 1953, US military casualties were transferred to MASHs further away. It was not said directly—the US officers were said to be far too polite to say it directly—but the chief of hospital, Egil Moe, had the clear impression that this was due to the fact that NORMASH had too many civilian patients, and that the hospital's reputation as a MASH had to be rebuilt.[112]

Caring for burn victims took more resources than NORMASH actually had. Wound care for one patient could take two doctors and two nurses an hour or more. During the hot season, wounds became colonized with maggots. Although this, in fact, promoted healing, the itching was intolerable for the patients. And for the nurses wound cleansing and bandaging became a difficult task.[113] Food was a limited resource: NORMASH got all its food from US supplies. This was for personnel and military patients. Koreans had to eat whatever was surplus to requirements. There were, in other words, several reasons why the number of civilians had to be limited.[114] But it was not easy to say "no." Children who had stepped on a mine or had been bombed by napalm needed professional healthcare. These conflicts between the dual missions of NORMASH continued throughout the war.

NORMASH also received prisoners of war (POWs). Like other patients, these men found a safe haven at the hospital. During the occupation of Norway, Germans had requisitioned parts of Norwegian hospitals. Nurses could not refuse to nurse German soldiers. In 1942 Gerd Semb had fled Norway to avoid nursing German soldiers, but as she said: "I can hate a system. But I can never bring myself to hate a person."[115] Such perspectives were also brought with nurses to NORMASH: when patients came to NORMASH, they were human beings rather than part of a system—individuals who required humanitarian service.

It was not only nurses with experience at hospitals who applied to serve at NORMASH. Nurses who had worked in China before the communist revolution also applied. Knowing the Chinese language was of great help. One sister mentioned this in particular when she applied for a new period in Korea in a letter to the matron-in-chief

> It has been peculiar to meet POW people. And it has been great fun to be able to speak to the Chinese prisoners. I feel so definitely that I am in the right place, and it's so strange feeling happy being able to give a little hand of help in a grey day. Again thank you, dear sister Ruth.[116]

Patients were first of all patients. Nurses triaging wounds did not also triage nationality. Only individual conditions counted when treatment was decided. Only after surgical treatment at the hospital and upon transportation to evacuation hospitals would POWs be sorted out and sent to a prison hospital near Pusan.

Blood transfusions were performed using blood from donors in the United States. Upon delivery in Korea, the blood was already between 10 and 14 days old and had to be used within a week. Bernard Paus commented:

> So it happens that in a MASH "a place in Korea" a friend or a foe, yellow, white or black patients are bedded side by side. Their lives are saved by half a litre of blood, voluntarily donated by an American man or woman living thousands of kilometres away.[117]

Some of the POWs were afraid of being poisoned by the Norwegian nurses. Propaganda had told them that they would be tortured and executed, or killed by stealth. Norwegian deacons and nurses who could speak Chinese and had worked as missionaries in China were of great help in translating and giving information about what was going on. Without such help, commencing anesthesia could be a problem. The medical condition was of course one thing, but the horror of believing that you were to be executed and would never wake up made patients fight back, trying to stay awake. A nurse who served in the second contingent later claimed that POWs, because they believed the propaganda, were often treated with greater care than allies. One of her POW patients had fought like a trapped wild animal at the beginning of narcosis: "I have seldom seen so much horror and anxiety as I saw in the eyes of that young man."[118] Inga Aardalsbakke sometimes had to taste the food or exchange the food with that of another patient before a POW dared to eat it. She claims that everybody was treated equally, no matter what his or her nationality or status.[119] A total of 172 POWs from North Korea and China received treatment at NORMASH.[120]

Some nurses at NORMASH appear to have made a deliberate choice to treat their work as a humanitarian rather than military endeavor. Their decision-making was independent of the expectations of their "commanding officers." Indeed, most did not even recognize the existence of a command structure apart from the nursing and medical hierarchies to which they were already accustomed. Their attachment to their own professional identity and their respect for their head nurse—"Sister Ruth"—engendered an independence and self-belief that seemed to insulate them from the politics of the Korean War medical services. In an account written several years after the war, Harda Hartvigsen, wrote in terms very similar to those of First World War civilian volunteer-nurse, Mary Borden, who had called her field hospital, "the second battlefield."[121] Hartvigsen's perspective evokes a similar image:

When the cannon roars at the front, and the fighting rages, the struggle inside the hospital continues, taking in its own particular form. At the front one thing is more important than anything else: to destroy the greatest number of human beings and munitions. Inside the hospital, we fight across a different front-line: we fight against death to preserve life. Neither nationality nor colour of skin matters. The only thing that matters is the Red Cross philosophy: "inter arma caritas: between the guns, love". Friend and foe get the same treatment. In fact, sometimes maybe a foe is nursed with greater care.[122]

The nurses took pleasure in their humanitarian service. Aslaug Hårvik wrote to Andresen on 29 September, 1951:

I feel the urge to thank you for granting me a place here. Thank you ever so much. We have a good time here—it is fun to see the people and the country, and feel the pleasure in helping soldiers, Koreans and our own people. It is no small thing to find happiness and pleasure in being one component in such a big work. I must express my heartfelt pleasure in this opportunity to serve others.[123]

In another letter, Ingrid Stafsnes declared: "we have all good things—and in addition, good humour. I must say again: 'I am glad to be alive.'" She added: "To be honest, I had imagined Korea, after all I have heard, to be a dreadful place . . . [But] I am in no way disappointed. On the contrary, I am grateful for this opportunity."[124]

The sense of the "thrill" of humanitarian service that resonates through the nurses' letters carries with it a strong element of personal power and autonomy. For some of these nurses, their work in Korea went well beyond "good nursing," and the experience was one they treasured. It was also an opportunity for learning. Stafnes wrote: "Heartfelt thanks for this opportunity to travel out here. It has been a great experience for me. I have learned a lot of things—not only nursing itself, but, perhaps even more, spiritual learning."[125]

These nurses do not come across as individuals who are "following orders." Although it was extremely rare for them to actively oppose any of the instructions they were given, most appear to have had a strong sense of their own priorities. Military casualties did take precedence at NORMASH; yet, the nurses' humanitarian instincts meant that the opportunity to assist any patient who arrived at their doors—whether military or civilian—was important to them.

Conflict of Leadership at NORMASH

Three Scandinavian countries had medical humanitarian missions in Korea. Sweden had an evacuation hospital in Pusan, Denmark a hospital ship,

Jutlandia; both kept their mission civil and under national control. Norway's mission, NORMASH was a Red Cross hospital under US command. Yet, although it became a military hospital, it struggled to be a military organization.

Insofar as it was under US command, it could be questioned whether NORMASH was under Norwegian national control at all. In an official letter, written before NORMASH officially opened, its first military commander had reported that the Norwegians had become popular with the US Army because they had agreed to serve close to the front lines of the war. It was observed that the Norwegians "don't play neutral as the Swedish are doing here."[126]

The question of whether this was a Norwegian or a US detachment was not easily settled. After a year's duty at the front, the commander of a later contingent reported that NORMASH did not have a flag that would show that this was an official Norwegian hospital. Not even the ensigns used on uniforms were Norwegian. He wanted a flag for use on parade, to demonstrate Norwegian sovereignty and create esprit de corps.[127] A flag was sent from Norway, but the ensigns used continued to be those of the US Army.

The transformation of the hospital from a Red Cross hospital to a military hospital, stationed close to the battle zone, caused misunderstandings on several levels. These related to the military status both of the hospital and of its personnel, although they do not appear to have influenced the medical treatment to any considerable extent. On November 1, 1951, the administration of NORMASH was transferred from the Norwegian Foreign Ministry to military command under the Norwegian Ministry of Defence. On a question from EUSAK about the status of the hospital, the answer was that the hospital was a military unit.[128] Even when it was a Red Cross hospital, it was for practical purposes considered part of the military and pragmatically adjusted to US military rules.[129] It was not communicated well in Norway that NORMASH was active in a war and a part of a UN Army.[130] The King of Norway, Haakon the Seventh, Commander in Chief of the Norwegian Armed Forces, addressed it as a Red Cross hospital in a telegram in 1952, something that the executive officer of NORMASH for that contingent, Major Steinum, found "offensive."[131]

The king was not the only person who mistook NORMASH for a civilian Red Cross hospital. A memorandum written at NORMASH and dated 1953, expressed concern about lack of information to the personnel. There were instances of conscious objectors and men who got the "unpleasant surprise" that life in a military camp was subject to military law and behavior. Meanwhile, commissioned officers described NORMASH as a "half-civil detachment."[132]

It was this half-civil status that had the most important implications in the organization of the hospital. A MASH was supposed to move on its own, and it was supposed to provide medical help for one particular army division.[133] NORMASH did support a division like the US MASHs, but it also operated as a Norwegian unit in a non-combatant role. This did from time to time cause friction between combatant officers and medical officers as combatant officers felt that medical officers interfered with tactical dispositions on how non-medical personnel should be used as guard soldiers. When questions were asked, the answer was that NORMASH was a hospital. Combatant officers were a support to the medical activity and the MASH was to be led by medical officers and not career officers. This arrangement may also have created a flatter structure between officers and soldiers than in US MASHs. The etiquette between officers and soldiers was said to be good but far too informal compared to the military conduct in an ordinary military detachment. This was a source of surprise to non-Norwegian visitors.[134] Peder Klingsheim was made a master sergeant. This rank was not in use in Norway—and so it did not mean much to him. Saluting was not so common, and he did not feel or think of himself as a soldier. He was a nurse in a hospital.[135]

Norway did not send Norwegian "orderlies" to serve in Korea. The first NORMASH contingent had only planned a staffing of 83 men in non-medical positions and for training to function as orderlies, and depended on employing Koreans in different positions. Eighty three men were too few to run a MASH properly. The US Army ordered a clearing company of 40 men and one officer together with an ambulance platoon to NORMASH. Some men in the clearing company were orderlies and were expected to work together with the nurses; but this proved to be a poor solution because of their limited training and their perspectives on military behavior. Norwegians had a more informal view about etiquette and more easy-going attitude toward military discipline than Americans.[136]

NORMASH: The Last Days

Norwegian nurses at NORMASH were not career officers. They were volunteer professional nurses. Their status as officers was temporary, though not without significance. In the last days of NORMASH there were incidents with the nurses where the question of whether this was a civil or a military hospital became important. It was only at this point, when the situation in Korea had changed from warfare to armistice, and the complement of patients had changed from combatant personnel to civilian Koreans, that a clash between the nurses and the chief of the hospital took place: nurses refused to attend roll call and parade after night duty. The chief of NORMASH wrote an angry letter to the Matron-in-Chief of the Army. He claimed that he, a civilian, tried to keep up a military appearance of the hospital, and demanded to know if the nurses were civilians or soldiers.[137] The Matron-in-Chief answered both wisely and diplomatically, showing a respect for both military rules and nurses' need for rest and sleep after night duty: "Yes. They are military and subjected to military law, but can't roll call be later in the day?"[138] The question was never raised again, but it symbolized the tensions inherent in the dual identity of NORMASH as both military and civil hospital.

After the armistice in July 1953, all military units were kept in a state of preparedness for further possible hostility. As the year passed it became clear that the armistice would endure. The patient flow at NORMASH changed during the last half of 1953. Combat wounds were no longer an issue. Still, patients with trauma from road accidents, accidental gunshot wounds, and mine injuries came to the hospital. In addition, there were somatic illnesses. These patients were not evacuated to the rear as before.

The tents were starting to wear out after over 2 years use—and, in any case, there was need for better conditions than the original structures could provide.[139] The operating theater, holding and postop tents were replaced with huts made of corrugated iron; and the bed capacity was increased from 60 to 90.[140] When NORMASH began functioning as a purely civil hospital, trauma surgery was not the primary demand. Koreans living in the area needed treatment for illnesses; such patients required longer hospital stays than those receiving stabilizing surgical treatments. With the end of hostilities, the supply of bank blood ceased. Staff at NORMASH established their own blood bank for Koreans; its donors were the Korean staff at NORMASH, and the first transfusions were done in March 1954.[141]

This new demand also led to changes for the nurses in their organization and work. Two theater nurses were reassigned to ward work. As the situation was stabilized, the Norwegian nurses started an outreach project to teach practical nursing in rural areas close to the hospital. This was also reflected in hiring practices: Korean nurses were employed and trained.[142] The original Norwegian idea of NORMASH—humanitarian aid to civilians and the development of Korea's own public health system—thus became more and more visible.

In 1951 there had been an agreement between Sweden, Denmark, and Norway that they would build a university clinic in Korea to aid education of health personnel.[143] During the war there had been discussions about whether NORMASH could be transformed into a university hospital in the event of a peace settlement in Korea.[144] After the armistice, the future use of the hospital again became an issue. Carl Semb, who had negotiated the first agreement for

Norway's participation in the UN army, again played a part. For Norwegians, there was a need for clarity. Should the hospital withdraw and be dismantled; or should it be converted into a joint Scandinavian university hospital? But an armistice is not a peace settlement. EUSAK wanted the Norwegian unit to retain its capacity for emergency response. And perhaps to flatter the Norwegians, the Chief Surgeon of EUSAK, General Smith, characterized NOR-MASH as the best of the six MASHs that had served at the front.[145]

NORMASH was kept at the front. But when EUSAK started to withdraw from the 38th parallel it lost the last remnants of its military purpose as an emergency response unit in case of renewed hostilities. There was no army to support. As the year went on, NORMASH was left—an outpost where there had once been a war. The first problem now was that there was no logistics chain left. Figures show that for the first half of 1954, 657 inpatients out of a total of 1,059 were civilians. Of 11,697 policlinic consultations, 5,956 were civilians, and the number of civilian patients was increasing.[146]

The Chief of the Hospital, Atle Berg, reported that NORMASH was not able to give adequate treatment to civilian patients. There were too few physicians, and the unit was equipped as a surgical hospital. A permanent hospital would have other medical issues and needs to deal with. The civilians' need for hospital services was huge, but it could not be fulfilled by NORMASH by August 1954.[147] And so, that autumn, the Norwegian field hospital was dismantled.

Conclusion

During the Korean War, Norway operated a hospital close to the battle zone, from July 1951 to October 1954. The NORMASH became a safe haven for different groups, including servicemen, POW, and civilians. When it was located at "The Orchard" it was seen by the nurses as a sanctuary that offered a place of safety away from the war. For wounded soldiers it was a military hospital where they could receive expert surgical and medical care; for other soldiers it was a place to make social calls and find friends; for some civilians it became a place to seek medical services; for others it offered a bed and work. One element of their professional independence was the camaraderie and cooperation shared by NORMASH nurses; another was their evident pride in their clinical skills. Beyond this, they appear to have shared a particular sense of purpose: they viewed their work at NORMASH as, at least in part, a humanitarian mission, operating alongside the treatment of wounded and sick combatants.

Approximately 90,000 patients were said to have been treated at NORMASH—in the wards and polyclinic.[148] The hospital served a military division like any other MASH at the front, but it never really became militarized. Uniforms and ranks were a matter of convenience. There were few women at the front. The nurse's rank was a protection against unwanted attention and gave authority to her orders in the hospital

Unlike the US MASHs, NORMASH was staffed by non-military personnel acting as volunteers. One of the main concerns of these volunteers was the wellbeing of the Korean civilians and their need for healthcare, food, and clothes. The nurses appear to have identified themselves as nurses giving humanitarian aid to a small country that was the victim of aggression, just as Norway had been during the invasion by Nazi Germany in 1940–1945. The Norwegian nurses at NORMASH—the "Korea sisters"—proved themselves valuable in a combat zone. Their professional skill and knowledge was commented-upon in the later memoirs of both doctors and patients. Although not specially trained as military nurses, they had confidence in their expertise, and were able to support patients with the most devastating of wartime injuries. And even in a time of war, they were able to run a hospital that many saw as a "sanctuary"—a safe haven providing not just treatment and nursing care to military casualties but also support, resources, respite, and friendship to Korean civilians.

NORMASH nurses interviewed for this study were proud of the humanity they had shown to both soldiers and civilians in Korea. Over 60 years after his service with NORMASH, nurse Peder Klingsheim said:

> When I look upon what we did for the Korean people in Korea, what it meant for them, and the friendships and bonds we forged with them, I think that we should never send soldiers to a conflict. We got the best result when we sent physicians and nurses.[149]

Klingsheim's words reveal the sense of humanitarianism that fuelled the work of NORMASH's nurses. They also suggest that such humanitarianism can act as a powerful source of energy and motivation driving a clinical mission. Although they rarely came into conflict with the military culture of their unit, the Norwegian nurses who served at NORMASH had their own sense of a purpose beyond military service—a humanitarian mission that gave them professional identity. Their personal agendas chimed well with the motto of the International Red Cross: "Inter Armas Caritas."

Notes

1. Trygve Lie, *Syv år for Freden* (Oslo: Tiden Norsk Forlag, 1954).
2. Carter Malkasian, *The Korean War 1950–1953* (Oxford: Osprey Publishing, 2001); Bruce Cummings, *The Korean War: A History* (New York: Modern Library, 2011).
3. Lars Bakke Asbjørnsen, *Fjellet med de Fallende Blomster—Skisser fra Korea* (Oslo: Forlaget land og kirke, 1952); Lorentz Ulrik Pedersen, *Norge i Korea. Norsk Innsats under Koreakrigen og Senere* (Oslo: C. Huitfeldt Forlag, 1991).
4. Knut Einar Eriksen and Helge Øystein Pharo, *Kald Krig og Internasjonalisering 1949–1965 Norsk Utenrikspolitisk Historie Bind 5* (Oslo: Universitetsforlaget, 1997); Nils A Røhne, *De Første Skritt inn i Europa. Norsk Europa-Politikk fra 1950* (Oslo: Institutt for Forsvarsstudier, 1989).
5. Eriksen and Pharo, *Kald Krig og Internasjonaliseing*; Kjetil Skongrand, *Norsk Forsvarshistorie Vol. 4. 1940–1970. Alliert i Krig og Fred* (Bergen: Eide forlag A/S, 2004).
6. Asbjørnsen, *Fjellet med de Fallende Blomster*; Pedersen, *Norge i Korea*; Finn Bakke, ed., *NORMASH—Korea i våre hjerter* (Oslo: Norwegian Korean War Veterans Association, 2010); Olav Sandvik, *Skjebnespill—Fra Kvinnherad til Vetrinærvesents Innside* (Oslo: Norsk Vetrinærhistorisk Selskap, 2012).
7. The Norwegian nurses' leader—Sister Ruth Andresen, encouraged her staff to write detailed letters about their experiences in Korea. These letters offer particularly vivid insights into the mentalities and lived experience of the Norwegian nurses: Box RAFA, File 3422, Letters to Matron-in-Chief, Forsvarets Sanitet 1952–1954, Riksarkivet, The National Archives of Norway, Oslo. Hereafter cited as Letters to Matron-in-Chief, Riksarkivet. In addition to the letters, another written source is of particular value: an unpublished account written by one of the nurses, Harda Hartvigsen, shortly after her experiences in Korea: Box RAFA, File 3422, Harda Hartvigsen, *Det Norske Feltsykehus i Korea og dets Arbeid Blant Sivilbefolkningen, Datert 15 September 1954*, Forsvarets Sanitet, 1954, Riksarkivet, The National Archives of Norway, Oslo. Hereafter cited as Hartvigsen, *Det Norske Feltsykehus i Korea*, Riksarkivet.
8. Five former nurses were interviewed specifically for this study. Whil acknowledging that this is a limited sample of the 111 nurses and 22 deacons who served, we would emphasize that the data produced, formed one of the study's most valuable and original elements. The participants were in their eighties and nineties when interviewed. All gave written consent for their testimony to be published. In each case, consent included the specification that their contribution should be attributed to them by name. They are: Gerd Semb, Inga Ardalsbakke, Kari Roll Kleppstad, Margot Isaksen, and Peder Klingsheim. The original, signed consent forms, along with the full transcripts of the interviews are stored securely at the Arctic University, Tromso, Norway, along with signed and dated permissions letters for the reproduction of the photographs reproduced in this article. The interviewing style was open and permissive, permitting participants to determine what was significant to them. The present study owes its central emphasis and its most original finding—the identification of NORMASH as a "sanctuary" and a humanitarian mission—in part, to the quality of its oral history interview data. The oral histories add complexity and nuance to the ostensibly "factual" information contained in the official record. Ethical approval for the study was granted by the Norwegian Social Science Data Services (NSD), and included permission for the naming of oral history interview participants at their own request, and for the publication of quotations from their interviews. Historians such as Paul Thompson,

Rob Perks, and Joanna Bornat, working mostly in a British context, advocate this approach as a means for capturing particular voices—most usefully those of individuals who had been silenced by their omission from the historical record: Paul Thompson, *The Voice of the Past: Oral History*, 3rd ed. (Oxford: Oxford University Press, 2000); Joanna Bornat and Rob Perks, *Oral History, Health and Welfare* (London: Routledge, 1991). More recently, scholars such as Geertje Boschma have done much to develop oral history methodology as an approach with particular relevance for historians of nursing: Geertje Boschma et al., "Community Mental Health Post-1950: Reconsidering Nurses' and Consumers' Identities," in *Routledge Handbook on the Global History of Nursing*, ed. Patricia D'Antonio, Julie Fairman, and Jean Whelan (New York: Routledge, 2013), 237–58. Barbra Mann Wall, Nancy E. Edwards, and Marjorie L. Porter, "Textual Analysis of Retired Nurses' Oral Histories," *Nursing Inquiry* 14, no. 4 (2007): 279–88.

9. Susan Armstrong-Reid and David Murray, *Armies of Peace: Canada and the UNRRA Years* (Toronto, Canada: University of Toronto Press, 2008).

10. Yihong Pan, "Never a Man's War: The Self-Reflections of the Women Soldiers of the New Fourth Army in the War of Resistance against Japan, 1937–45," *Research on Women in Modern Chinese History/Jindai Shongguo Funu Shi Yanjiu* 24 (2014): 83–131. We are deeply indebted to Yihong Pan for forwarding us a full copy of the original, English version of her paper (which was translated into Chinese for publication)

11. On the concept of "agency" in historical work, see also: J. L. Lee, "Patient/Client Agency in American Nursing, 1900–1986" (PhD diss., University of Southern California, 1988); Annie Devenish, "Performing the Political Self: A Study of Identity Making and Self-Representation in the Autobiographies of India's First Generation of Parliamentary Women," *Women's History Review* 22, no. 2 (2013): 280–94; Manuela Scarci, *Creating Women: Representation, Self-Representation, and Agency in the Renaissance* (Toronto, Canada: Centre for Reformation and Renaissance Studies, University of Toronto, 2013); Chris Pearson, "Dogs, History and Agency," *History and Theory* 52 (2013): 128–45; David Gary Shaw, "The Torturer's Horse: Agency and Animals in History," *History and Theory* 52 (2013): 146–67. See also Charlotte Epstein, "Theorizing Agency in Hobbes's Wake: The Rational Actor, the Self, or the Speaking Subject?" *International Organization* 67 (2013): 287–316.

12. Iain Gordon and Lifeline, *A British Casualty Clearing Station on The Western Front 1918* (Stroud: The History Press, 2013); Henry Owens, *A Doctor on the Western Front: The Diary of Henry Owens 1914–1918* (Barnsley: Pen & Sword Books Ltd., 2013); Mark Harrison, *The Medical War: British Military Medicine in the First World War* (Oxford: Oxford University Press, 2010); Christine E. Hallett, *Containing Trauma: Nursing Work In The First World War* (Manchester: Manchester University Press, 2009); Christine E. Hallett, *Veiled Warriors: Allied Nurses of the First World War* (Oxford: Oxford University Press, 2014), 67–54; John Stevens and Caroline Stevens, eds., *Unknown Warriors. The Letters of Kate Luard RRC and BAR, Nursing Sister in France 1914–1918* (Stroud: The History Press, 2014).

13. Scott Christopher Woodard, "The Story of the Mobile Army Surgical Hospital," *Military Medicine* 168 (July 2003): 503–13; Sanders Marble, "Forward Surgery and Combat Hospitals: The Origin of the MASH," *Journal of the History of Medicine and Allied Sciences* 69, no. 1 (May 2012): 68–100.

14. Booker King and Ismalil Jatoi, "The Mobile Army Surgical Hospital (MASH): A Military and Surgical Legacy," *Journal of The National Medical Association* 97, no. 5 (May 2005): 648–56.

15. Woodward, "The Story of the Mobile Army Surgical Hospital," 503.

16. King and Jatoi, "Mobile Army Surgical Hospital," 656.

17. Quincealea Brunk, "Nursing at War: Catalyst for Change," *Annual Review of Nursing Research* 15 (1997): 217–36.

18. Mary T. Sarnecky, *A History of the U.S. Army Nurse Corps* (Philadelphia: University of Pennsylvania Press, 1999), 310–11.

19. Margaret G. Blake, "With the Army Nurse Corps in Korea," *The American Journal of Nursing* 51, no. 6 (1951): 387; Anonymous, "With the First MASH," *The American Journal of Nursing* 51, no. 6 (1951): 386.

20. Jill E. McNair, *A British Army Nurse in The Korean War* (Stroud: Tempus Publishing, 2007).

21. Eric Taylor, *Wartime Nurse: One Hundred Years from The Crimea to Korea 1854–1954* (London: Robert Hale Ltd., 2001), 192–207.

22. Frances Omori, *Quiet Heroes: Navy Nurses of the Korean War 1950–1953 Far East Command* (Saint Paul: Smith House Press, 2000).

23. Michael S. Baker, "Military Medical Advances Resulting from the Conflict in Korea, Part 1: Systems Advances That Enhanced Patient Survival," *Military Medicine* 177 (2012): 423–29; Bernhard Paus, "Kirurgiske erfaringer fra Det norske feltsykehus i Korea," *Nordisk medicin* 51, no. 11 (1954): 384–88.

24. Martin Sæther, *Over Alle Grenser. Norges Røde Kors 100 år* (Oslo: Aschehoug & Co, 1965).

25. Eldrid Mageli, *Med rett til å hjelpe. Historien om Norges Røde Kors* (Oslo: Pax Forlag, 2014).

26. Sæther, *Over Alle Grenser*; Magne Brekken, "Humanitær bekymring og militær begeistring: Norske beretninger fra balkankrigene 1912–1913" (Masters diss., Norwegian University of Science and Technology, Trondheim, 2006); Harald Natvig, *Fra den finske frihed krigen I 1918: Vestarmeen* (Kristiania: Mittet, 1918); Monica Janfelt, "Ambulan-shjälp till Finland 1918: Nordisk Röda Kors-aktion mellan privat och offentlig nödhjälp," in *Den privat-offentliga gränsen. Det sociala arbetets strategier och aktörer i Norden 1860–1940*, ed. Janfelt Monica (København, Denmark: Nordisk Ministerråd, 1999), 301–26; Gunnar Ulland, *Under Genferkorset i Etiopia: Med den norske ambulance* (Oslo: Aschehoug, 1936); Mageli, *Med rett til å hjelpe*; Kaare Gulbransen, *Gull og grønne skoger* (Bergen: J.W. Eides Forlag, 1956).

27. Torstein Dale, *Det Norske Feltsykehus i Korea. NORMASH 1951–1954* (Oslo: Forsvarets Sanitet, 1955); Ole J. Malm, *Forsvarets Sanitet. 50 Ar Under Felles Ledelse. 1941–1991* (Oslo: Forsvarets Overkommando, 1991); Kaare Granå, *Hærens sanitet 1888–2002* (Oslo: Forsvarets Sanitet with InfoMediaHuset AS, 2004); Sæther, *Over Alle Grenser*.

28. Kjetil Skogrand, "Norge og Koreaspørsmålet, 1945–1953," (Masters diss., The University of Oslo, 1994).

29. Gulbransen, *Gull og grønne skoger*, trans. Jan-Thore Lockertsen, 343.

30. Hallvard Tjelmland, *Den kalde krigen* (Oslo: Det Norske Samlaget, 2006); Skogrand, *Norsk Forsvarshistorie*; Olav Njølstad, *Jens Chr. Hauge—Fullt og helt* (Oslo: Aschehoug, 2008).

31. Lie, *Syv år for freden*, 311.

32. Skogrand, *Norge og Koreaspørsmålet*.

33. Njølstad, *Jens Chr. Hauge—Fullt og helt*.

34. Sten Florelius, *Rapport fra Norges Røde Kors til Utenriksdepartementet* (Oslo: The Norwegian Red Cross, 1952).

35. Box RAFA, File 3422, T. Dale. Militære Grader for Personellet ved Norsk Feltsykehus til Korea av 25.04.51, Forsvarets Sanitet 1951, Riksarkivet, The National Archives of Norway, Oslo.

36. Box RAFA, File 3422, Kingdom of Norway and the United Stated of America. Agreement Between The Government of Norway and The United States of America Concerning the Participation of a Norwegian Mobile Surgical Hospital in The United Nations Operations in Korea, 17 September, 1951, Forsvarets Sanitet 1951, Riksarkivet, The National Archives of Norway, Oslo.

37. Ibid.

38. F. Otto Apel and Pat Apel, *MASH—An Army Surgeon in Korea* (Lexington: The University Press of Kentucky, 1998); Albert E. Cowdry, *The Medics' War* (Honolulu: University Press of the Pacific, 2005), 180.

39. Box RAFA, File 3422, Arne Hvoslef, Report to Surgeon General Norwegian Armed Forces Medical Services, of November 17, 1951, Forsvarets Sanitet, 1951, Riksarkivet. The National Archives of Norway, Oslo.

40. Apel and Apel, *Mash—An Army Surgeon in Korea*.

41. Florelius, *Rapport fra Norges Røde Kors*; Dale, *Det Norske Feltsykehus i Korea*, 67–68.

42. Ruth Andresen, *Fra Norsk Sanitets Historie—Kvinners Innsats i Militær Sykepleie* (Oslo: NKS-Forlaget, 1986).

43. Ole Georg Moseng, *Framvekst og profesjonalisering—Norsk Sykepleierforbund gjennom 100 år (1912–2012) Bind 1* (Oslo: Akribe AS, 2012).

44. Birgit Evensen, *Fra Sykehusloftet til MH-Bygget: Sykepleierutdanningens Historie i Tromsø* (Tromsø: Eureka Forlag, 2003).

45. Malm, *Forsvarets Sanitet. 50 Ar under Felles Ledelse*.

46. Andresen, *Fra Norsk Sanitets Historie*.

47. Olav Sandvik, *Skjebnespill: Fra Kvinnherad til Vetrinærvesents Innside*; F. Bakke, *NORMASH—Korea i Våre Hjerter* (Oslo: Norwegian Korean War Veterans Association, 2010), 16.

48. Box RAFA, File 3422, Anonymous Report Dated 10 April, 1951, Forsvarets Sanitet, 1951, Riksarkivet, The National Archives of Norway, Oslo.

49. Dale, *Det Norske Feltsykehus i Korea*; Bakke, *NORMASH—Korea i Våre Hjerter*, 14–16.

50. Rønnaug Wüller, "Med Norsk Feltsykehus til Korea," *Sykepleien: Organ for Norsk sykepleierforbund* 39 (March 1952): 126–32; Gerd Semb, Oral History, January 8, 2011, conducted by Jan-Thore Lockertsen, Lørenskog, Norway. Herafter cited as Gerd Semb, Oral History.

51. Margot, Isaksen, Oral History, November 27, 2013, conducted by Jan-Thore Lockertsen, Greverud, Norway. Hereafter cited as Margot Isaksen, Oral History.

52. K. E. Van Buskirk, "The Mobile Army Surgical Hospital," *The Military Surgeon* 113 (July/December 1953): 29.

53. Box RAFA, File 3422, Heide Inga Stamnes, Letter/Report to Matron-in-Chief, Forsvarets Sanitet 1954, Riksarkivet, The National Archives of Norway, Oslo.

54. Inga Årdalsbakke, Oral History, December 7, 2011, conducted by Jan-Thore Lockertsen, Skei, Norway. Hereafter cited as Inga Årdalsbakke, Oral History.

55. Isaksen, Oral History.

56. Bernhard Paus, "Medisinsk Liv ved den Koreanske Krigsskueplass," *Tidsskrift for den Norske Lægeforening* 74, no. 1 (January 1954): 11–15.

57. Deborah L. Hallquist, "Development in the RN First Assistant Role During the Korean War," *AORN Journal* 10 (2005): 644–47.

58. Brunk, "Nursing at War: Catalyst for Change," 217–36. See also Sarnecky, *A History Of the U.S. Army Nurse Corps.*

59. Sarnecky, *A History Of the U.S. Army Nurse Corps*, 289, 305.

60. Peder, Klingsheim, Oral History, January 28, 2015, conducted by Jan-Thore Lockertsen, Askøy, Norway. Hereafter cited as Peder Klingsheim, Oral History. Klingsheim was educated between 1948 and 1952, 3 years training as nurse and an additional year in social and theological training.

61. Box RAFA, File 3422, R. Andresen, Letter from Matron-in-Chief to Chief of Staff, September 12, Fortsvarets Sanitet, 1951, Riksarkivet, The National Archives of Norway, Oslo.

62. Klingsheim, Oral History.

63. Box RAFA, File 3422, Arne Hvoslef. Report to The Surgeon General, The Norwegian Armed Forsces Medical Services, November 17 1951, Forsvarets Sanitet, 1951, Riksarkivet. The National Archives of Norway, Oslo. Quotation translated by Jan-Thore Lockertsen.

64. Ibid.

65. Box RAFA, File 3422, T. Dale, Report from General Surgeon, The Norwegian Armed Forsces Medical Services to Ministry of Defense December 10, Forsvarets Sanitet, 1951, Riksarkivet. The National Archives of Norway, Oslo.

66. Letters to Matron-in-Chief, Riksarkivet.

67. Box RAFA, File 3422, Finn Backer, Response of The Royal Ministry of Defence to The General Surgeon, The Norwegian Armed Forces Medical Services, 15 December, Forsvarets Sanitet, Oslo.

68. Dale, *Det Norske Feltsykehus i Korea.*

69. Hartvigsen, *Det Norske Feltsykehus i Korea*, Riksarkivet.

70. Ibid.

71. Box RAFA, File 3422, Herman, Ramstad, Report, June 9, 1951 for The Norwegian Red Cross, June 9, 1951, Forsvarets Sanitet, 1951, Riksarkivet, The National Archives of Norway, Oslo.

72. Box RAFA, File 3422, T. Dale, Letter written by Surgeon General of Norwegian Armed Forces Medical Services to The Norwegian Red Cross, October 20, 1951, Fortsvaret Sanitet, 1951, Riksarkivet, The National Archives of Norway, Oslo.

73. Ragnar W. Nilssen, *Med Røde Kors i Korea* (Stavanger: Misjonsselskapets forlag, 1952).

74. Sæther, *Over Alle Grenser*; Janfelt, "Ambulanshjälp till Finland 1918," 301–26.

75. James Jacobs, *From the Imjin to the Hook: A National Service Gunner in the Korean War* (Barnsley: Pen & Sword Books Ltd., 2013), 66.

76. Colin Baker, *Wild Goose: The Life and Death of Hugh Van Oppen* (Cardiff: Mpemba Books, 2002); See also Arvid Fjære, "Vaktsoldat i NORMASH," in *NORMASH—Korea i Våre Hjerter*, ed. F. Bakke (Oslo: Norwegian Korean War Veterans Association, 2010), 21–25.

77. Klingsheim, Oral History. Quotation translated by Jan-Thore Lockertsen.

78. Isaksen, Oral History.

79. Thor Treider, "Fra Vinterkrigen til Korea," in *I krig for fred*, ed. Haakon Bull-Hansen (Oslo: Kagge forlag, 2008), 55.

80. Gerd Semb, Oral History. Quotation translated by Jan-Thore Lockertsen.

81. Ibid.

82. E. Lund, "Sykepleierskene i Moderne Krig. Beskyttelse Gjennom Militære Grader og Uniform Absolutt Nødvendig," *Adresseavisen* 186, no. 10 (January, 1952): 5.

83. Box RAFA, File 3422, Carl, Semb. Report Number Three to The Ministry of Defence, Norway, Forsvarets Sanitet, 1951, Riksarkivet. The National Archives of Norway, Oslo. On atrocities committed during the Korean War; see Philip D. Chinnery, *Korean Atrocity!Forgotten War Crimes 1950–1953* (Barnsley: Pen & Sword Books Ltd., 2009).

84. Box RAFA, File 3422, H. Ramstad, Report to The Norwegian Red Cross, dated June 9, 1951, Forsvarets Sanitet, 1951, Riksarkivet. The National Archives of Norway, Oslo; Box RAFA, File 3422, C. Semb, Report Number Four to the Ministry of Defence, Forsvarerts Sanitet, 1951, Riksarkivet, The National Archives of Norway, Oslo.

85. Box RAFA, File 3422, Erling Hjort, Instructions/Standing Orders for Nurses, August 1952, Forsvarets Sanitet, 1952, Riksarkivet, The National Archives of Norway, Oslo.

86. Asbjørnsen, *Fjellet med de Fallende Blomster*, 15.

87. Unni Foss, "Over til Korea," in *Norge i Korea. Norsk Innsats under Koreakrigen og Senere*, ed. L. U. Pedersen (Oslo: C. Huitfeldt Forlag A.S, 1991), 49–52.

88. Gulbransen, *Gull og Grønne Skoger*.

89. K. Skogrand, "Norge og Koreaspørsmålet 1945–1953," (Masters diss., The University of Oslo, 1994).

90. Gerd Semb, Oral History Interview.

91. Pedersen, *Norge i Korea*.

92. Gerd Semb, Oral History Interview.

93. Bernhard Paus Falck, Private Diary, transl. Lucie, Paus, Falk, Author's own collection (Jan-Thore Lockertsen). Quotation translated by Lucie Paus Falck.

94. Nilssen, *Med Røde Kors i Korea*.

95. Gulbransen, *Gull og grønne skoger*.

96. Wüller, "Med norsk feltsykehus til Korea," 126–32.

97. Lund, "Sykepleierskene i moderne krig."

98. Lucie Paus Falck, Oral History, January 9, 2015, conducted by Jan-Thore Lockertsen, Oslo, Norway. Hereafter cited as Lucie Paus Falck, Oral History. Lucie Paus Falck is the daughter of the late Bernard Paus. After the war, she followed her father to Seoul, Korea, and worked, between 1958 and 1960, at the National Medical Center (NMC). NMC was a joint venture between Norway, Denmark, and Sweden, to educate and train Korean health personnel. It was handed over to South Korea in 1968.

99. Gerd Semb, Oral History Interview.

100. Box RAFA, File 3422, Report of April 25, 1951, Forsvarets Sanitet, Riksarkivet. The National Archives of Norway, Oslo. Quotation translated by Jan-Thore Lockertsen.

101. Box RAFA, File 3422, Ruth Andresen, "Norske sykepleiersker i Korea," Account, May 4, 1954, Riksarkivet. The National Archives of Norway, Oslo.

102. Evlyn, Nilssen, Letter, March 23, 1953, Letters to Matron-in-Chief, Riksarkivet. Quotation translated by Jan-Thore Lockertsen.

103. Pedersen, *Norge i Korea*.

104. Box RAFA, File 3422, Erling Falsen Hjort,Report from Hjort toThe General Surgeon, The Norwegian Armed Forces Medical Services, Forsvarets Sanitet, 1952, Riksarkivet. The National Archives of Norway, Oslo; Box RAFA, File 3422, Petter Sundt. Letter to The General Surgeon, The Norwegian Armed Forces Medical Servicses of 28 June, Forsvarets Sanitet, 1952, Riksarkivet. The National Archives of Norway, Oslo.

105. Box RAFA, File 3422, T. Dale. Letter from The General Surgeon, The Norwegian Armed Forces Medical Services to Chief of Hospital NORMASH, Hjort, of July 19, 1952, Forsvarets Sanitet, 1952, Riksarkivet. The National Archives of Norway, Oslo.

106. Box RAFA, File 3422, Ingrid, Stafnes. Letter to Matron-in-Chief, Ruth Andresen, March 20, 1953, Forsvarets Sanitet, 1953, Riksarkivet. The National Archives of Norway, Oslo. Hereafter cited as Stafnes, Letter to Matron-in-Chief, Riksarkivet.

107. Fjære, "Vaktsoldat i NORMASH," 21–25.

108. Nilssen, *Med Røde Kors i Korea.*

109. Hartvigsen, *Det Norske Feltsykehus i Korea*, Riksarkivet.

110. Box RAFA, File 3422, R. Andresen, Report from Head Nurse, NORMASH, to The General surgeon, The Norwegian Armed Forces Medical Services, July 5, 1952, Forsvarets Sanitet, 1952, Riksarkivet. The National Archives of Norway, Oslo. Hereafter cited as Andresen, Report from Head Nurse, July 5, 1952, Riksarkivet.

111. Stafnes, Letter to Matron-in-Chief, Riksarkivet.

112. Box RAFA, File 3422, Egil Moe, 1953. Report from Chief of Hospital, NORMASH, to The General Surgeon, Norwegian Armed Forces Medical Services, May 8, 1953, Forsvarets Sanitet, 1953, Riksarkivet. The National Archives of Norway, Oslo.

113. Hartvigsen, *Det Norske Feltsykehus i Korea*, Riksarkivet.

114. Andresen, Report from Head Nurse, July 5, 1952, Riksarkivet.

115. Gerd Semb, Oral History Interview. Quotation translated by Jan-Thore Lockertsen.

116. Box RAFA, File 3422, Aslaug Hårvik, Letter to Matron-in-Chief of September 29, 1951, Forsvarets Sanitet, 1951, Riksarkivet. The National Archives of Norway, Oslo. Hereafter cited as Hårvik, Letter to Matron-in-Chief, Riksarkivet. Quotation translated by Jan-Thore Lockertsen.

117. B. Paus, "Feltsykehuset i Korea," *Aftenposten* 92, no. 464 (October 8, 1951). Quotation translated by Jan-Thore Lockertsen.

118. Hartvigsen, *Det Norske Feltsykehus i Korea*, Riksarkivet. Quotation translated by Jan-Thore Lockertsen.

119. Årdalsbakke, Oral History.

120. Dale, *Det norske feltsykehus i Korea.*

121. Mary Borden, *The Forbidden Zone* (London: William Heinemann Ltd., 1929).

122. Hartvigsen, *Det Norske Feltsykehus i Korea.*

123. Hårvik, Letter to Matron-in-Chief, Riksarkivet. Quotation translated by Jan-Thore Lockertsen.

124. Stafsnes, Letter to Matron-in-Chief, Riksarkivet.

125. Ibid.

126. Box RAFA, File 3422, Hans Sollie, Report to Major Volckmar, the Norwegian Korea Office of June 27, 1951, Forsvarets Sanitet, 1951, Riksarkivet, The National Archives of Norway, Oslo. Quotation translated by Jan-Thore Lockertsen.

127. Box RAFA, File 3422, Karl Petter Steinum, Report to The General Surgeon, The Norwegian Armed Forces Medical Services, from Administration Officer NORMASH, October 7, Forsvarets Sanitet, Riksarkivet, The National Archives of Norway, Oslo.

128. Box RAFA, File 3422, Finn Backer. The Royal Ministry of Defense to the Norwegian Royal Foreign Ministry July 3, 1952, Forsvarets Sanitet, 1952, Riksarkivet, The National Archives of Norway, Oslo.

129. Box RAFA, File 3422, Arne Hvoslef, Letter to The General Surgeon, The Norwegian Armed Forces Medical Services, 20 October 1952, Forsvarets Sanitet, 1952, Riksarkivet, The National Archives of Norway, Oslo.

130. Florelius, *Rapport fra Norges Røde Kors*.

131. Box RAFA, File 3422, K. P. Steinum, Report from Administration Officer, NORMASH, to The Norwegian Armed Forces Medical Services, August 31, 1952, Forsvarets Sanitet, Riksarkivet, The National Archives of Norway, Oslo.

132. Box RAFA, File 3422, Otto Krogh-Sørensen, Report from Administration Officer, NORMASH, to The Norwegian Armed Forces Medical Services, January 9, 1953, Forsvarets Sanitet, 1953, Riksarkivet, The National Archives of Norway, Oslo.

133. Woodard, "The Story of the Mobile Army Surgical Hospital," 503–13.

134. Box RAFA, File 3422, E. Moe. Report from Chief of Hospital, NORMASH, to The General Surgeon, The Norwegian Armed Forces Medical Services, May 8, 1953, Forsvarets Sanitet, 1953, Riksarkivet, The National Archives of Norway, Oslo.

135. Klingsheim, Oral History Interview.

136. Box RAFA, File 3422, H. Ramstad, Report from Chief of Hospital, NORMASH, to Surgeon General, Norwegians Armed Medical Services, Forsvarets Sanitet, 1951, Riksarkivet, The National Archives of Norway, Oslo.

137. Box RAFA, File 3422, Atle Berg. Military Discipline for Nurses at The Field Hospital: Enquiry from Chief of Hospital, NORMASH, to Matron-in-Chief, The Norwegian Armed Forces Medical Services, July 29, 1954, Forsvarets Sanitet, 1954, Riksarkivet, The National Archives of Norway, Oslo.

138. Box RAFA, File 3422, R. Andresen. Military Discipline for Nurses at The Field Hospital: To Chief of Hospital, NORMASH, August 7, 1954, Forsvarets Sanitet, 1954, Riksarkivet, The National Archives of Norway, Oslo. Quotation translated by Jan-Thore Lockertsen.

139. Box RAFA, File 3422, Egil Thoresen.Report from Chief of Hospital, NORMASH, to Surgeon General, Norwegian Armed Medical Services October 28, Forsvarets Sanitet, 1953 Riksarkivet, The National Archives of Norway, Oslo.

140. Box RAFA, File 3422, Ragnar Nordlie, Report from Chief of Hospital, NORMASH, to The General Surgeon, The Norwegian Armed Forces Medical Services, March 5, 1954, Forsvarets Sanitet, 1954, Riksarkivet, The National Archives of Norway, Oslo.

141. Box RAFA, File 3422, Ragnar Nordlie. Report from Chief of Hospital, NORMASH, to The General Surgeon, The Norwegian Armed Forces Medical Services, of April 7, 1954, Forsvarets Sanitet, 1954, Riksarkivet, The National Archives of Norway, Oslo.

142. Ibid.

143. Nilssen, *Med Røde kors i Korea*.

144. Box RAFA, File 3422, T. Dale, From Surgeon General, The Norwegian Armed Forces Medical Services to the Royal Ministry of Defence, page 2, Forsvarets Sanitet, 1953, Riksarkivet, The National Archives of Norway, Oslo.

145. Box RAFA, File 3422, C. Semb, To The Ministry of Defence: Further use of NORMASH after the armistice, of 3 November, Forsvarets Sanitet, 1953, Riksarkivet, The National Archives of Norway, Oslo.

146. Box RAFA, File 3422, B. Paus, The Norwegian Field Hospital in Korea: On closure or not, August 23, 1954, Forsvarets Sanitet, 1954, Riksarkivet, The National Archives of Norway, Oslo.

147. Box RAFA, File 3422, A. Berg, Chief of Hospital, NORMASH, to The General Surgeon, The Norwegian Armed Forces Medical Services: On Closure of NORMASH, of August 31, 1954, Forsvarets Sanitet, 1954, Riksarkivet, The National Archives of Norway, Oslo.

148. Dale, *Det norske feltsykehus i Korea*.

149. Klingsheim, Oral History Interview. Quotation translated by Jan-Thore Lockertsen.

Disclosure. The authors have no relevant financial interest or affiliations with any commercial interests related to the subjects discussed within this article.

JAN-THORE LOCKERTSEN, RN
Lecturer in Theatre Nursing
UiT –The Arctic University of Norway
Tromso, Norway

ÅSHILD FAUSE, RN, PhD
Asc. Professor of Nursing
UiT –The Arctic University of Norway
Tromso, Norway

CHRISTINE E. HALLETT, RGN, PhD
Professor of History
The University of Huddersfield
United Kingdom

THE ROLE OF PLACE IN THE HISTORY OF NURSING

Introduction

BARBRA MANN WALL
University of Virginia

In 2009, Patricia D'Antonio called for a consideration of place as a category for analysis in nursing history. Focusing on nursing as a practice discipline in a global arena, she suggested more scholarship that crosses linguistic, geographical, and cultural boundaries.[1] Along these lines, the articles in this series serve as entry points into interdisciplinary debates about the importance of place in local and regional histories of nursing. Funded by the Virginia Foundation for the Humanities, the Southern Association for the History of Medicine and Science, and the American Association for the History of Nursing, the authors in this study assert that regional interactions can provide insights into understanding national and global developments, while at the same time contributing to a more diverse history of nursing. We ask: what is place and how can we better understand it as a concept of analysis? How can an understanding of place help nurses to begin to think about connections between their work and local and regional histories? To what extent are particular histories of nursing place based?

As Martha Howell and Walter Prevenier assert today, "historians treat a much greater range of topics, and they do so by employing a much wider variety of theories and methods." This change has occurred as historians have encountered other disciplines and have taken their "tools, method, theory, and subject matter" to enhance understanding of their own areas of study.[2] We bring together theoretical discussions from geographical studies, history, and

Nursing History Review 28 (2020): 127–132. A Publication of the American Association for the History of Nursing. Copyright © 2020 Springer Publishing Company.
http://dx.doi.org/10.1891/1062-8061.28.127

sociology to obtain insights into varied approaches to think about how a focus on place might provide new insights into the history of nursing. Authors have been invited to select an area of their research in the form of a short paper that engages at some level with the concept of place.

In their book, *The Power of Place: Bringing Together Geographical and Sociological Imaginations*, political geographer John A. Agnew and cultural geographer James S. Duncan assert the centrality of place to geography and history. They theorize, "Places provided both the real, concrete settings from which cultures emanated to enmesh people in webs of activities and meanings and the physical expression of those cultures in the form of landscapes."[3] As well, "place, both in the past and in the present . . . serves as a constantly re-energized repository of socially and politically relevant traditions and identity."[4] Other authors expand on the meaning of place. Historical geographer Denis Cosgrove, for example, asserts that places as physical locations are permeated with "human meaning." Place is not only a site for habitation, but it must also "possess significance for people."[5] Similarly, geographer Tim Cresswell defines place as "a meaningful location" to which "people are attached . . . in one way or another."[6]

We build on these ideas by employing Agnew's framework of three aspects of place: physical locations or regions; locales or settings where social interactions occur as people go about living their lives; and a sense of place, or how people affectively identify with a place.[7] We assert that a focus on place enables us to understand multiple meanings about nursing in multiple contexts. Different elements of place are considered: regions such as segregated Virginia; locales where nurses work, such as intensive care units; and places such as hospitals and military bases where social interactions engendered specific identities and race and class dynamics.[8]

Case studies in this series address the history of nursing in three areas of the southern United States: Washington, DC, Virginia, and Maryland, the latter centering on Baltimore. This is not an argument for exceptionalism. Rather, the writers ask: what is it about place that allows us to rethink key questions in nursing history? While the geographic proximity of these areas is clear, each case sees the notion of place in different ways.

Lourdes Carhuapoma demonstrates the power of place at a specific hospital where nurses worked—Johns Hopkins Hospital—where interdisciplinary approaches combined to create a specialty area in nursing. She focuses on the crucial role of place in the training of nurses who shaped the care of the sickest of neurosurgical patients beginning in 1923 at Johns Hopkins Hospital in Baltimore, Maryland. This place was the premier teaching institution in the country, where both clinical facilities and the medical school were linked. As early as the 1880s and 1890s, the Johns Hopkins Hospital led the nation in specialty training in eye and ear diseases, skin problems, children's diseases, genito-urinary conditions, disorders of the nervous system, and surgery. In 1889, the School of Nursing began under the leadership of Isabel Hampton, followed by Adelaide Nutting and Lavinia Dock.[9] Harvey Cushing was at Johns Hopkins Hospital when he published his 1905 paper, "The Special Field of Neurological Surgery."[10] Thus, the creation of a specialty for neurological nursing at Hopkins is not surprising. Indeed, Hopkins served as a place for new social and professional interactions to occur.

Victoria Tucker illustrates contested meanings of place through the examination of a black nurse who entered a place presumed to be white, a school of nursing in Virginia during the transition from segregation to desegregation on college campuses and in healthcare facilities. As a case study, she examines the educational and professional life of Mavis Claytor, the first black woman to graduate from the University of Virginia School of Nursing. Even though, through a blind review process, the School of Nursing accepted Claytor into the program, the attendant at the nurse's dormitory denied her a room. Indeed, a black body in a place assumed to be white was considered incompatible with the racial norms of the day—long-held beliefs that a black person would not have the intelligence to get a baccalaureate degree in nursing. Claytor's specific experience in nursing school can be seen, in part, as a reflection of her location in Virginia during desegregation. But why Virginia? It embodied the advances, resistance, and setbacks of segregation/desegregation that were happening across the country. In thinking about Virginia, Edmund S. Morgan's argument is key: In any history of southern places, one must consider the "central paradox of American history": the "marriage of slavery with freedom." To Morgan, "the key to the puzzle, historically," lies in Virginia. As the nation was forming, Virginians owned more than 40% of the slaves. Four of the first five presidents were from Virginia and were all slaveholders.[11] Most of the tobacco, the most valuable crop in early America, came from Virginia. As Tucker argues, Virginia's history also is situated in places such as Jamestown, where English men and women first settled and decided to grow tobacco with labor impressed upon others; and Monticello, where Thomas Jefferson, over his lifetime, enslaved up to 400 laborers, 130 at any given time.[12] Yet the prominence of these people and places overshadows other histories, particularly those of black women who had to overcome the power of place—with prejudice and Jim Crow segregation—to become nurses. A focus on black nurses as a case study reveals how place is not finite: Southern heritage both persisted and changed in the last half of the 20th century.

A different way to examine place is through the interactions it can produce as a sense of place—the attachments people have to a place. Reynaldo Capucao Jr., mines new insights into the understandings of how nurses experienced place through his study of Filipino nurses in Hampton Roads, Virginia, since 1965. He discusses the relationship between labor migration and naval establishments, which became critical centers for place-making and community development for Filipinos. What sets Hampton Roads apart is that it is the largest naval station in the world, Naval Station Norfolk, with the most numerous Filipino population on the East coast. Capucao understands place not only as a location but also as a sense of place where social and cultural conflict occurred. His history is one forged within a context of imperialism in the late 19th century. After 1965, however, place and circumstance combined to signal a major transformation of the nursing workforce when skilled nurses migrated to the United States as wives of Filipino service members who had been recruited into the U.S. Navy. Capucao's study is of particular interest because he links American military and nursing recruitment policies to Hampton Roads, which contributed to the Filipino diaspora around the state and country. Since the 1930s, a shortage of nurses has loomed over the nursing profession in the United States. During the latter half of the 20th century, one solution the country implemented was the importation of internationally educated nurses (IENs). By 1989, 73% of the IEN workforce were Filipino nurses. At the same time, interactions among diverse groups of people produced specific class and ethnic identities. While Hampton Roads' naval base fostered a vibrant Filipino nursing community, it also contributed to new class dynamics in nursing and challenged old black/white dichotomies.

The final case study expands on the importance of place as an institution where the practice of nursing occurred. Trina Kumodzi examines the emergence of trauma nursing at the University of Maryland Shock Trauma Unit (STU) in the 1970s and 1980s. The STU became a specific locale where practices, negotiations, and relationships gave rise to a new specialty—the trauma nurse. Kumodzy grounds her study in a particular geographic location, the industrial, post-automobile city of Baltimore in the second half of the 20th century. As Agnew argues, however, social worlds "cannot be completely understood apart from the macro-order of location and the territorial identity of a sense of place."[13] Thus, from a new perspective, Kumodzy shows how the trauma unit allows us to understand the many elements of place, not only as a specific geographic location but also as a locale where social relations developed among physicians and nurses within a specific site. She begins with a discussion of the rapid expansion of urban places such as Baltimore after World War I, when millions of people from the rural South moved to cities further north and west. This had a huge impact on available healthcare resources and coincided as hospitals expanded into classrooms for medical students, where the poor became teaching subjects. Over the 20th century, like other large cities, Baltimore became a site for increased urban violence and traffic accidents, and patients became ever more available for hospital teaching in the 1970s when the STU was established. Kumodzy asserts that in establishing such a place, certain histories are privileged, that is, that of physicians; yet nurses also had a large role to play in creating the STU.

As nursing history expands its interdisciplinary collaborations, it is useful to think about how elements of place can be considered in our work. The papers in this series invoke the meaning of place from different perspectives, with the premise being that there are many ways that recognize place as a powerful tool to think about our work. Examining its different meanings helps us to think about core issues in nursing history such as specialization, diversity in education, nurse migration, and social and institutional struggles structured by race, class, and ethnicity. By being sensitive to place, historians can better understand the rich contexts needed for analysis of these important topics in nursing history. As well, writing about place allows dissemination of local and regional histories in ways that recover new voices and insights previously hidden to nurses and historians.[14]

Notes

1. Patricia D'Antonio, "Thinking about Place: Researching and Reading the Global History of Nursing," *Texto Contexto-Enferm* 18, no. 4 (October/December 2009): 766-772. doi:10.1590/S0104-07072009000400019.

2. Martha Howell and Walter Prevenier, *From Reliable Sources: An Introduction to Historical Methods* (Ithaca, NY: Cornell University Press, 2001). First quotation is on page. 143; second is on page. 144.

3. John A. Agnew and James S. Duncan, eds., *The Power of Place: Bringing Together Geographical and Sociological Imaginations* (London: Routledge, 1989), vii.

4. Agnew and Duncan, *The Power of Place*. Quotation is on page. 7.

5. Dennis Cosgrove, "Power and Place in the Venetian Territories," in *The Power of Place: Bringing Together Geographical and Sociological Imaginations*, eds. John A. Agnew and James S. Duncan (London: Routledge, 1989), 194.

6. Tim Cresswell, *Place: An Introduction* (Chichester: Wiley Blackwell, 2015). Quotation is on page 12.

7. John A. Agnew, *Place and Politics: The Geographical Mediation of State and Society* (Abingdon: Routledge, 2015).

8. J. Nicholas Entrikin, "Place, Region, and Modernity," in *The Power of Place: Bringing Together Geographical and Sociological Imaginations*, eds. John A. Agnew and James S. Duncan (London: Routledge, 1989), 30–43.

9. Mame Warren, ed., *Our Shared Legacy: Nursing Education at Johns Hopkins, 1889–2006* (Baltimore: Johns Hopkins University Press, 2006).

10. Harvey Cushing, "The Special Field of Neurological Surgery," *Bulletin of the Johns Hopkins Hospital* 16, no. 168 (1905): 77.

11. Edmund S. Morgan, *American Slavery, American Freedom* (New York: W.W. Norton & Co, 1975), 4–5.

12. Kevin R. Hardwick and Warren R. Hofstra, *Virginia Reconsidered: New Histories of the Old Dominion* (Charlottesville: University of Virginia Press, 2003), 1. See also Alan Taylor, "Hero or Villain, Both and Neither: Appraising Thomas Jefferson, 200 Years Later," *UVA Magazine* 107, no. 4 (Winter 2018): 48–51.

13. Agnew, *Place and Politics*, 2.

14. Charles W. J. Withers, "Place and the 'Spatial' Turn in Geography and in History," *Journal of the History of Ideas* 70, no. 4 (October 2009): 637–658. doi:10.1353/jhi.0.0054.

Disclosure. The author has no relevant financial interest or affiliations with any commercial interests related to the subjects discussed within this article.

Barbra Mann Wall, PhD, RN, FAAN
University of Virginia
225 Jeanette Lancaster Way
Charlottesville, VA 22903

Matriarchs of the Operating Room: Nurses, Neurosurgery, and Johns Hopkins Hospital, 1920–1940

Lourdes R. Carhuapoma
University of Virginia

> On one day a poor scrubwoman lies before you on the operating table; the next perhaps a Cardinal who has travelled across a continent to seek relief at the far famed Johns Hopkins Hospital. You who have served in operating rooms know the story. If you feel from what I have said that our services are different from your own, come to see us. An exchange of ideas will be refreshing and helpful to us both.[1]

These were the words of Agnes Doetsch, a leader in surgical nursing at Johns Hopkins Hospital and the School of Nursing in the early 20th century. Written in 1935 and entitled, "Speaking of Operating Rooms," she was referring to those who traveled far and near to "seek relief" at the famed hospital. Her words serve as an example of the power of place as a site where an "exchange of ideas" could occur, where heightened vigilance and care could be carried out regardless of social class, and where a specialized team of nurses and physicians could come together in a neurosurgical unit.

This historical study demonstrates the power of place at a specific locality—Johns Hopkins Hospital in Baltimore, Maryland—where interdisciplinary approaches combined to create a specialty area in nursing in 1923. The study is not meant to devalue the many interpretations of nursing in specific hospitals.[2] Rather, it takes a different perspective to discuss the institution of Johns Hopkins Hospital itself, nurses' roles in creating a neurosurgical specialty practice, and the conditions at Hopkins that made it possible for nurses and patients to thrive.

By the early 20th century, Johns Hopkins Hospital was the premier teaching institution in the country, where both hospital clinical facilities and the medical school were linked. Harvey Cushing was an associate

Nursing History Review 28 (2020): 133–142. A Publication of the American Association for the History of Nursing. Copyright © 2020 Springer Publishing Company.
http://dx.doi.org/10.1891/1062-8061.28.133

professor in surgery at Hopkins when he published his 1905 paper, "The Special Field of Neurological Surgery,"[3] seen as the "foundation document of neurosurgery's development over the century."[4] As early as the 1880s and 1890s, the Johns Hopkins Hospital had led the nation in specialty training in eye and ear diseases, skin problems, children's diseases, genito-urinary conditions, disorders of the nervous system, and surgery. Other famous physicians such as William S. Halsted, William H. Welch, and William Osler were at Hopkins. Osler, in particular, valued nurses in their roles in saving lives.[5] It is not surprising, then, that the beginning of units specifically designed to care for critical neurosurgical patients began at a place such as Hopkins. It helped shape the training of nurses in the early 20th century to provide intensive care to the most complex of neurosurgical patients. Clearly this is a study about an elite institution, which has its drawbacks. Yet elite institutions such as Hopkins fed into other schools of nursing and helped set standards elsewhere.

Background

Quaker philanthropist Johns Hopkins established the hospital in 1889 in Baltimore, Maryland, and in his original plans he had included a nursing school.[6] Thus, in April of 1889, the School of Nursing opened under the leadership of Isabel Hampton and eventually Mary Adelaide Nutting and Lavinia Dock. It was at Hopkins that these nursing leaders established a tradition of leadership in the field. They advocated that nursing required not only character but also knowledge and judgment.[7] Over the next several years, the nurse training program became the model for the training of nurses in the United States.

The evolution of intensive care units in the United States has been discussed by Julie Fairman, Joan Lynaugh, and Arlene Keeling. From them we learn that advances in medical technology, treatments, and an overall understanding of critical illness led to the need for the sickest of patients to be cared for in a centralized location by physicians and nurses trained to tend to the seriously-ill.[8] Although the literature centers on the birth of intensive care units in the 1950s and 1960s, the first known neurosurgical recovery room where patients received specialized intensive nursing care dates back to the 1920s at Johns Hopkins Hospital.

Yet the specialty of neurological nursing began earlier. In 1887, physician Charles Karsner Mills wrote *The Nursing and Care of the Nervous and Insane*.[9] The emergence of wards specializing in the care of patients with neurological illnesses began in the early 1900s with the creation of the New York

Neurological Institute in 1909. One of the founders of the Institute, Joseph Collins, wrote about the need for the specialized training of nurses in the care of patients with neurological disorders. Published in 1911 in the *American Journal of Nursing*, he emphasized the need for the additional training of nurses in neurological nursing; and a course on care of patients with nervous disorders, did, in fact, result.[10]

In 1912, Nutting, the former superintendent of nurses and principal of the training school at Johns Hopkins Hospital, wrote her classic manuscript for the United States Bureau of Education, entitled *Educational Status of Nurses.*[11] At the time of publication, nursing had rapidly advanced to the state of a profession that required regulatory efforts for training and maintaining a skilled and proficient workforce. Thirty states, including Maryland, had adopted laws informing adequate preparation of professional nurses. Many other states were expected to do the same in the next coming years. Also by then, more than 1,000 training schools had been established in the United States with 30,000 students in attendance.[12] Thus, the need developed to provide general guidance in the form of regulation to oversee the training of nurses. Elite programs, such as the Johns Hopkins Hospital Training School for Nurses, led in highlighting novel concepts in the training of professional nurses.[13]

One example was the specialized training of faculty in the nurse training program. Nutting wrote:

> In a very few schools higher standards of teaching and a better quality of work are secured through the introduction of specially trained teachers. Among the schools which have established such teaching positions are those belonging to the Johns Hopkins Hospital at Baltimore, the Massachusetts General Hospital at Boston, and St. Luke's, the Presbyterian, and Bellevue Hospitals, in New York.[14]

In addition to the specialized training of instructors, Nutting believed that institutions offering varied clinical experiences for nurses were well-positioned to better prepare students for the role of the professional nurse. She asserted:

> The ability of the hospital to give a thorough and complete training in nursing rests then mainly upon two conditions: First, the character, variety, and extent of its service; second, the state of its finances. The first condition determines whether or not it affords suitable and sufficient opportunities for instruction and training; the second indicates its ability to provide suitable instructors, equipment, accommodation for students, and other appurtenances of a school.[15]

Johns Hopkins Hospital met these criteria. As Rosemary Stevens notes, the support of the Flexner Report of 1910, the connection of the hospital and the medical school, and the creation of a novel nurse training program helped the hospital to become the premier medical center in the country. By 1911, the hospital maintained 300 beds and 145 nursing students, and instructors received specialized training in the education of professional nurses. While larger institutions existed, Hopkins was also sizable and provided a vast array of clinical opportunities for nursing students, given its position as a leader in advances in medicine and surgery.[16]

Neurosurgical Nursing as a Specialty

Lewellys Baker, Physician in Chief at Hopkins, supported the specialization of nurses as early as 1912. Nutting quoted him:

> Thus far, nurses have, for the most part, been content to be general practitioners of nursing, but already some have begun to specialize, and it needs only half an eye to see that the near future will be marked by an extension of this tendency to specialization in nursing. While each nurse should have a general training in fundamentals of the art, there is no reason why she should not, like the physician, choose some one particular field of work which appeals to her interest and for which her natural talents may make her especially suitable. The time is fast approaching when we shall have nurses who attend chiefly or solely to obstetrical cases, others who care only for pediatric cases, only for nervous and mental cases, only for fever cases, only for operative cases, only for metabolic cases, etc. Nurses who desire successfully to specialize will be compelled to acquire unusual training and experience, just as is the medical specialist.[17]

In the late 19th and early 20th centuries, the field of surgery at Johns Hopkins Hospital experienced tremendous growth. Discoveries in neuroanatomy and neuropathology advanced, which led Cushing to create the neurosurgical specialty at the Johns Hopkins Hospital beginning in the 1890s. The specialty grew over the first two decades of the 20th century.[18] William Halsted, surgeon-in-chief, developed a revolutionary postgraduate residency program in surgery, the first of its kind in the United States.[19] While residents trained in all fields of surgery, subspecialties burgeoned as the role of the generalist diminished.[20]

In 1910, Walter Edward Dandy graduated from the Johns Hopkins School of Medicine. Following the completion of his medical degree, Dandy pursued his surgical residency at Johns Hopkins Hospital and completed his training in 1919.[21] Neurosurgical procedures were becoming increasingly more complicated, requiring a highly-skilled surgical team to attend to such cases. Dandy was a pioneer in the many advances in neurosurgery, as well as the training of a proficient and skilled team to assist in performing highly complex cases. Dandy and his team, for example, discovered the intricacies of the circulation of cerebrospinal fluid and the causes of hydrocephalus, ventriculography, and pneumoencephalography.[22]

In 1920, an article in the *American Journal of Nursing* carefully detailed the significance of nursing on the postoperative care of neurosurgical patients. Gertrude Dwyer, from the Neurological Institute of New York, wrote, "It is essential that nurses desiring to specialize in this work should have had previously a good general surgical training and we would advise also a special study of the anatomy and physiology of the brain and spinal cord."[23] Dwyer's work supported the emergence of a dedicated specialty area in nursing; emphasized the collaborative efforts between physicians and nurses; and highlighted the autonomy of nurses required in the care of neurosurgical patients. She wrote:

> Perhaps in no branch of medicine can a nurse be so helpful to a physician as in the care of brain cases. I want to impress upon my readers the absolute necessity of observing carefully each patient, in order that no transient incident of the illness may be lost to the physician in charge. Be no longer automatons, 'mere makers of beds and dispensers of drugs,' but active allies of the medical profession, keenly alive to the changes taking place in your patients. The clue in any case may be a fleeting description, a temporary weakness in a limb, a slight convulsion, a sensation of tingling in the hand or foot, a blurring of vision, a transient diplopia, a change in the mental state, irrelevant remarks, etc. The apparently insignificant things must be recorded and reported.[24]

Thus, while nurses were to be "helpful" to physicians, they were also to be "active allies" with them.[25] Nurses implemented Dwyer's dictums in the vast and diverse clinical experiences in the field of neurosurgery available at Hopkins.

Nancy Weyland McClung Gravett graduated from the Hopkins nurse training program in 1921. While a student, she meticulously documented her clinical experiences in the operating room along with her learning of anatomy and physiology. She carefully noted findings that indicated an abnormality in patients. Regarding injury to the skull, she wrote: "Bleeding from nose, ears, etc. to be noticed . . . white fluid from ear—cerebrospinal fluid—is a pathognomonic sign of injury to base of skull. Do not stop up the ear but allow the fluid to flow out."[26] Indeed, nurses had great responsibility that required advanced learning about the needs of neurosurgical patients. Their knowledge afforded patients greater protection in an environment that was constantly changing.

The Brain Team

In the early 20th century, as neurosurgery expanded, the operating room became an ever important place for expert care. At that time, the training of surgical nurses at the Johns Hopkins Hospital Training School for Nurses became a collaborative effort between physicians and nurses, and a brain team developed. The curriculum for nurses consisted of a combination of didactic and clinical training. Students could observe surgical operations first hand while also participating in a practical component of formal instruction in the surgical clinic setting. House surgeons gave lectures on specific conditions and students then demonstrated the nursing care. For example, Warfield Firor, Dandy's surgical resident, gave lectures for the surgical nursing course while a nurse led the clinical instruction.[27]

In 1922, Dandy became chief neurosurgeon at the Johns Hopkins Hospital. The same year, he recognized the need for heightened vigilance in the immediate postoperative care of neurosurgical patients.[28] Thus in 1923, Firor and he created a special place dedicated for attention to the sickest of neurosurgical patients who required intensive monitoring during this crucial postoperative period.[29] In the years following, units designed to care for either neurosurgical or neurological patients developed throughout the country.[30] The emergence of large-scale combined neurosurgical and neurological intensive care units in academic centers developed primarily in the late 1970s through the 1980s, although evidence supports the development of a combined unit in the late 1950s at Mayo Clinic—St. Mary's Hospital in Rochester, Minnesota.[31]

A. McGehee Harvey, in *Adventures in Medical Research: A Century of Discovery at Johns Hopkins*, fluently describes the neurosurgical recovery room that Dandy created.

The design included a floorplan with specific connections between the operating and recovery rooms. He wrote:

> It is noteworthy that perhaps the first organized unit was the postoperative recovery room adjacent to the old operating room in the Johns Hopkins Hospital, where neurosurgical patients were cared for around the clock by a special nursing group prior to returning to their rooms. It was located on the fourth floor of the old Surgical Building and consisted of three beds. This was in 1923 during the period July 5, 1923 – January 29, 1925 when Warfield M. Firor was Dandy's resident surgeon. When the Halsted and Carnegie buildings were built, the neurosurgical recovery room was moved to Halsted 7. It was the nearest room to the operating room and was adjacent to the doctors' quarters.[32]

Significantly, Harvey added, "It was staffed twenty-four hours a day with special recovery room nurses. This was the beginning of careful attention to airway care, temperature control, circulatory monitoring, fluid and electrolyte balance and observation of the state of consciousness of the patient."[33]

In this defined geographic area of the hospital, the recovery room was an extension of the operating room, which indicated a continuum of care by staff intimately familiar with the operative details of the case at hand. Nurses trained so they could provide the vigilance necessary to tend to such patients. Indeed, it was the nursing care that defined the intensity of the recovery room environment. The model continued into the 1940s as evidenced by the writings of Hugo Rizzoli, Dandy's surgical resident. He wrote: "All patients were taken to this unit after surgery to recover from anesthesia, and when conscious and alert, they moved to their respective rooms. More seriously-ill patients with craniotomies were observed in this unit 1 or more days until they became stable. There was a nurse in each of these two adjacent rooms continuously—day and night."[34]

Elizabeth Wallace Sherwood came to Johns Hopkins Hospital in 1924 as General Operating Room Supervisor. She received her diploma in nursing from New York City Hospital in 1918, followed by time at Teachers College at Columbia University and work at Henry Street Settlement until 1919. The following years she held the positions of Operating Room Assistant Supervisor in two New York area hospitals before assuming the supervisory role at Johns Hopkins Hospital.[35] In her role, Sherwood displayed power and authority in regulating the daily activities in the spaces of the operating rooms.

Rizzoli defines the role of the operating room supervisor as a "matriarch." He wrote, "The resident would stand above the patient, sponge stick in hand, ready to scrub the operative area at exactly 8:00 a.m. The matriarch supervising the OR apparently had the power to determine this time."[36] The matriarch's command of place was clear: she ensured that the operating room functioned with a distinct level of organization and precision.

Another important nurse was Agnes Doetsch, who eventually became Dandy's longtime surgical scrub nurse. She had demonstrated interest in the physical sciences prior to a career in nursing. After earning a baccalaureate degree from Goucher College in 1921, Doetsch served in a number of roles. She was a Laboratory Assistant in Biology at Eastern High School in Baltimore, and she completed coursework at the Marine Biological Laboratory, Cold Spring Harbor, in Long Island. She pursued graduate work in Botany at Johns Hopkins and then served as an Instructor in Physics and Biology at Western High School in Baltimore. In 1927, she enrolled in summer coursework at Columbia University's Teachers College, and in 1931 received a diploma in nursing from the Johns Hopkins Hospital School of Nursing. She eventually became Head Nurse of the Halsted Surgery Clinic and in 1936 received the appointment of Instructor at the Johns Hopkins Hospital School for Nurses.[37]

In her 1935 publication, "Speaking of Operating Rooms," Doetsch described the physical space of the operating room and the neurosurgical recovery room:

> There is one other room, no. 725, set aside for nasal and dental work and two small dressing rooms intended originally as recovery rooms for neurosurgical patients but, since the opening of the Halsted Clinic and its neurosurgical ward with a connecting bridge between the operating room and the ward, these patients are now sent back to the ward.[38]

Doetsch eloquently described her thoughts on the nursing profession: "As nurses, I think we are justified in feeling that nursing skill, like the skill that lies in the fingers, eyes and brain of the surgeon can be developed into an art, in other words, that nursing is an art as well as a profession."[39]

Conclusion

Nurses such as Sherwood and Doetsch displayed significant power and influence in their respective roles as leaders in neurosurgical nursing in the early 20th century at Johns Hopkins Hospital. Their instruction of "intelligent postoperative care" led to the continuation of an effective model in which neurosurgical patients underwent a successful recovery due to the careful monitoring of nurses with specialized training.[40] The recovery room became a significant place where nurses had an enhanced capacity for observing patient's conditions.

This article has discussed the forces that came together to remake the space of the hospital to include a distinct unit for recovery of neurosurgical patients. Nurses' and doctors' successes were the results of a highly-skilled, reputable surgical team trained in a premier institution. With the assistance of his ever-efficient and well-trained brain team, Dandy performed over 1,000 neurosurgical cases annually.[41] By 1940, his brain team consisted of five nurses, two of whom were nurse anesthetists, in addition to his surgical residents, intern, orderly, and secretary.[42] The nursing contribution to the creation and advancement of the first neurosurgical recovery room at Johns Hopkins Hospital was crucial. Conditions at Hopkins in the early 20th century helped make their work possible.

Notes

1. Agnes Doetsch, "Speaking of Operating Rooms," *The Alumnae Magazine of The Johns Hopkins Hospital School of Nursing* 34, no. 1 (January 1935): 12–16, in the Alan Mason Chesney Medical Archives of the Johns Hopkins Medical Institutions, Baltimore, Maryland (hereafter cited as Alan Mason Chesney Medical Archives). Quotation is on p. 16.

2. For information on education at Johns Hopkins, see Mary Carol Ramos, "The Johns Hopkins Training School for Nurses: A Tale of Vision, Labor, and Futility," *Nursing History Review* 5 (1997): 23–48; and Mame Warren, ed., *Our Shared Legacy: Nursing Education at Johns Hopkins, 1889–2006* (Baltimore: Johns Hopkins University Press, 2006).

3. Harvey Cushing, "The Special Field of Neurological Surgery," *Bulletin of the Johns Hopkins Hospital* 16, no. 168 (1905): 77.

4. Samuel H. Greenblatt, "The Special Field of Neurological Surgery," *Neurosurgery* 57, no. 6 (December 2005): 1075.

5. For general histories of hospitals, see Charles E. Rosenberg, *The Care of Strangers: The Rise of America's Hospital System* (New York: Basic Books, 1987), 206; and Gunther Risse, *Mending Bodies, Saving Souls: A History of Hospitals* (New York: Oxford University Press, 1999).

6. John Shaw Billings, "The Plans and Purposes of the Johns Hopkins Hospital," *The Medical News*, May 11, 1889, accessed December 11, 2018, https://books.google.com/books?hl=en&lr=&id=b3lxNQbpbfsC&oi=fnd&pg=PA1&dq=billings+the+plans+and+purposes+of+johns+hopkins+hospital&ots=cgdPfjd5TV&sig=PZb_U6id-b9PS3srb3lYjkGpm_Q#v=onepage&q=billings%20the%20plans%20and%20purposes%20of%20johns%20hopkins%20hospital&f=false

7. Warren, *Our Shared Legacy*.

8. Julie Fairman and Joan Lynaugh, *Critical Care Nursing: A History* (Philadelphia, PA: University of Pennsylvania Press, 1998); see Arlene W. Keeling, "Blurring the Boundaries between Medicine and Nursing: Coronary Care Nursing, Circa the 1960s," *Nursing History Review* 12 (2004): 139–164.

9. Charles Karsner Mills, *The Nursing and Care of the Nervous and the Insane* (Philadelphia, PA: J.B. Lippincott Co., 1887); See Jeanette C. Hartshorn, "Aspects of the Historical Development of Neuroscience Nursing," *Journal of Neuroscience Nursing* 18, no. 1 (1986): 45–48, for further discussion.

10. Joseph Collins, "Nursing in Nervous Diseases First Paper: The Teaching in Neurological Hospitals," *American Journal of Nursing* 11, no. 6 (1911): 434–439.

11. M. Adelaide Nutting and U.S. Bureau of Education, *Educational Status of Nursing Bulletin, No. 7* (Washington, DC: Government Printing Office, 1912).

12. Ibid.

13. Ramos, "The Johns Hopkins Training School for Nurses"; Warren, *Our Shared Legacy*.

14. Nutting, *Educational Status*, 7.

15. Ibid., 18.

16. Rosemary Stevens, *American Medicine and the Public Interest* (New Haven, CT: Yale University Press, 1971), Updated with new Introduction, Berkeley: University of California Press, 1998.

17. Nutting, *Educational Status*, 10.

18. Stevens, *American Medicine*.

19. Irving J. Sherman, Ryan M. Kretzer, and Rafael J. Tamargo, "Personal Recollections of Walter E. Dandy and His Brain Team," *Journal of Neurosurgery* 105, no. 3 (2006): 487–493.

20. Stevens, *American Medicine*.

21. Hugo V. Rizzoli, "Dandy's Brain Team," *Clinical Neurosurgery* 32, no. 1985, 23–37.

22. Walter E. Dandy and Kenneth D. Blackfan, "An Experimental and Clinical Study of Internal Hydrocephalus," *Journal of the American Medical Association* 61, no. 25 (1913): 2216–2217; Roderick L. Tondreau, ""Ventriculography and

Pneumoencephalography: Contributions of Dr. Walter E. Dandy," *RadioGraphics* 5, no. 4 (July 1985): 553–555; and Sherman et al., "Personal Recollections."

23. Gertrude M. Dwyer, "Nursing Care Following Operations on Brain and Spinal Cord," *American Journal of Nursing* 20 (1920): 613–617. Quotation is on p. 613.

24. Ibid., 616.

25. Ibid.

26. Nancy Wayland, Student Notebooks, Class of 1921, Nancy Wayland McClung Gravatt Collection, 511882, Alan Mason Chesney Medical Archives.

27. "The Johns Hopkins Hospital School of Nursing Circular of Information 1936–1937." The Johns Hopkins Hospital School of Nursing Institutional Records 1928–1945, Box 2, Alan Mason Chesney Medical Archives.

28. A. McGehee Harvey, *Adeventures in Medical Research: A Century of Discovery at Johns Hopkins* (Baltimore and London: The Johns Hopkins University Press, 1974); See also Eelco F. M. Wijdicks et al., "The Early Days of the Neurosciences Intensive Care Unit," *Mayo Clinic Proceedings* 86, no. 9 (2011): 903–906.

29. Harvey, *Adventures in Medical Research*.

30. Hartshorn, "Aspects of the Historical Development of Neuroscience Nursing."

31. Wijdicks et al., "The Early Days of the Neurosciences Intensive Care Unit"; and Arlene Keeling, *The Nurses of Mayo Clinic: Caring Healers* (Rochester, MN: Mayo Clinic, 2014).

32. Harvey, *Adventures in Medical Research*, 65.

33. Ibid.

34. Rizzoli, "Dandy's Brain Team," 26.

35. "The Johns Hopkins Hospital School of Nursing Circular of Information."

36. Rizzoli, "Dandy's Brain Team," 26.

37. "The Johns Hopkins Hospital School of Nursing Circular of Information."

38. Doetsch, "Speaking of Operating Rooms," 16.

39. Ibid., 12.

40. "The Johns Hopkins Hospital School of Nursing Circular of Information."

41. Sherman et al., "Personal Recollections."

42. Rizzoli, "Dandy's Brain Team;" Sherman et al., "Personal Recollections,"

Disclosure. The author has no relevant financial interest or affiliations with any commercial interests related to the subjects discussed within this article.

LOURDES R. CARHUAPOMA, RN, MS, ACNP-BC, CCRN
University of Virginia School of Nursing

Race and Place in Virginia: The Case of Nursing

Victoria Tucker
University of Virginia

This article examines contested meanings of place through a case study of the educational and professional life of Mavis Claytor, the first black woman to graduate from the University of Virginia School of Nursing.[1] It does so within the context of entrenched racialized legislation and geographically-based socio-cultural norms, as academic and healthcare centers in Virginia transitioned from segregation to desegregation in the 1950s through the 1980s. The article seeks to understand how and why Virginia became a national site for the massive resistance movement that countered school desegregation; and how, within this context, Claytor made sense of place as she entered newly-integrated programs and spaces in Virginia. History as place reveals how local nurses' work connects to where they lived, studied, and practiced, providing a renewed lens for analysis in nursing history.

Virginia: A Place of Analysis

Black nurses' concept of place in America is manifold, and history provides a lens for illuminating this meaning. Black nurses' experiences cannot be understood without considering the intricate interworking of American history (colonialization, slavery, Jim Crow laws, massive resistance) and acknowledging Virginia's central lineage within this narrative. While Virginia shares many features with other states, it also has a distinct identity as the site where slavery began in the United States.[2] Historical context is situated in places such as Jamestown, where enslaved Africans grew tobacco in colonial settlements; in Richmond's Lumpkin Jail, where enslaved blacks were either held, traded, or severely punished[3]; and in Charlottesville's Monticello, Thomas Jefferson's plantation, where he enslaved approximately 400 laborers at this plantation site across his lifespan.[4] Indeed, Jefferson's *Notes on the State of Virginia*,

Nursing History Review 28 (2020): 143–157. A Publication of the American Association for the History of Nursing. Copyright © 2020 Springer Publishing Company.
http://dx.doi.org/10.1891/1062-8061.28.143

written approximately a decade after the Declaration of Independence, made his views known that blacks were intellectually inferior to whites, "in endowments both of body and mind."[5] In 1819, Jefferson founded the University of Virginia as a segregated institution for white men. Relevant history is also present in Virginian places such as Hampton, where northern and southern black nurses studied and mastered nursing practice at the segregated Hampton Training School for Nurses, known as Dixie Hospital Training School; in Roanoke, where black nurses learned and cared for black patients in the black-established health infrastructure known as Burrell Memorial Hospital; and in Charlottesville, where black licensed practical nursing students studied at Jackson P. Burley High School and practiced at the University of Virginia Health System. Additionally, Piedmont Sanatorium in Burkeville trained black nurses and provided tuberculosis care for black patients in Virginia from 1918 through the 1960s.[6] Virginia continues to be a physical and intellectual incubator of American political and social movements. A detailed exploration of black nurses in Virginia not only brings a new lens to an underexplored area of nursing history, but it can also help dismantle discriminatory policies and practices from which health disparitites arose.

Place: A Lens for Analysis

Historians Katherine McKittrick and LaKisha Michelle Simmons' works illuminate the complex meanings surrounding place through their analysis of black women's geographies.[7] McKittrick, for example, argues that:

> The geographic meaning of racialized human geographies is not so much rooted in a paradoxical description as it is a projection of life, livability, and possibility. Poetics, real and imagined geographies, put demands on traditional geographic arrangements because they expose the racial-sexual functions of the production of space and establish new ways to read (and perhaps live) geography.[8]

In her book, *Demonic Grounds: Black Women and The Cartographies of Struggle*, McKittrick prioritizes black women's humanity and disrupts stagnant depictions and understandings of black women's geographies and their movement within real and imagined spaces. McKittrick unveils the shifting relationships between the places black women claim, celebrate, create, negotiate, occupy, protect, and infiltrate.

Simmons' study of black women in New Orleans affirms McKittrick's work and is particularly helpful as she describes place in the context of segregation. In *Crescent City Girls: The Lives of Young Black Women in Seg-regated New* Orleans, Simmons asserts, "Figuring out one's place was made more difficult by the fact that spaces and the meanings associated with them, though seemingly self-evident and stable, were never fixed."[9] Her description of fluidity has present-day relevance when studying desegregation of Virginia nurse training programs and healthcare settings. Simmons discussion on place challenges the observer to acknowledge the vast meanings associated with the concept.

To examine place in segregated settings, it is also essential to understand how law and nursing interacted. Two landmark federal decisions were crucial in granting black nurses and nursing students access to academic, professional, and clinical sectors. The 1954 Supreme Court ruling *Brown v Board of Education*, led by lawyers and members of the National Association for the Advancement of Colored People (NAACP), banned segregation within education systems. The 1964 Civil Rights Act's Title VI ended sanctioned institutional segregation and discrimination in public spheres. Access, however, did not insulate blacks from racism, discriminatory practices, or segregationist symbols. Black nurses navigated both integration's visible paths and segregation's prominent shadows.

Black Nurses' Identity in the United States

Black women were caregivers and healers during slavery in America.[10] Yet nursing history records often begin with the development of professional nursing institutions and at the nexus of credentialing, a metric that has often cast the white nurse as the only nurse worthy of historical merit. A deeper understanding of segregationist and exclusionary practices provides context for this gap. Black nurses predominately had three options in the early 1950s: apply to a licensed practical nursing program, a historically black professional nursing program, or apply to a nursing school that accepted black students under the restriction of quotas.[11] Black nurses and nursing students found themselves bolstered between systemic oppression and a generational lineage of civil rights pursuits between the 1950s and 1980s. During this time, black nurses and nursing students sought to advance their professional identity and strategically address the health inequalities in the black community.[12]

Claytor came of age in the Jim Crow South during the 1950s and 1960s. At that time, discriminatory and segregationist practices in the United States perpetuated disparate health outcomes in the black community.[13] National mortality and morbidity statistical comparisons between black and white citizens in the 1950s unveiled a haunting actuality surrounding the falsehood of "separate but equal"; it was in fact "separate but deadly."[14] Leslie A. Falk, physician and professor at Meharry Medical College, documented evidence of health disadvantages in the 1966 publication, "The Negro American's Health and the Medical Committee for Human Rights." Falk inquires:

> How do health and medical care fit into this scheme of things? First, let us review some of an extensive literature on the Negro's health status. Mortality statistics are almost universally adverse when Negro and white rates are compared. The average U.S. Negro dies seven years earlier than the average U.S. white. In the South, a Negro male has a particularly short life expectancy—only 50 years, compared with 67 for the white male.[15]

Statistical data use grew expeditiously between 1890 (the first census conducted by the US government) and 1950. Instituted reports such as the *Vital Statistics of the United States*, a national report that the US Department of Health, Education, and Welfare published, included population data collected during the 60-year period. The 1950 report, for example, included data about fetal, infant, and population mortality, showing lacks with large discrepancies compared to whites.[16] Statistical data revealed numbers and comparison of racial groups over time, yet analysis did not acknowledge segregation or the black community's unequal access to quality healthcare. Black healthcare professionals and other activists independently and collectively organized to disrupt the segregated medical and education system of the Jim Crow era; and black nurses, in particular, remained at the center of health and community activism.

Virginia's Recalcitrance to Racial Integration: Massive Resistance

Black women's fundamental human and civil rights, such as education, survival, privacy, and pleasure predicated upon a sophisticated understanding and adept navigation of the contractual nature of segregated and integrated spaces. Claytor was born into a close-knit family in 1943 to Lucy Smith Claytor. One of seven children, she and her family grew up in Callaway, Virginia, a town located in rural Franklin County. Her roots in this area are both deep and wide; she is the granddaughter of Wyatt Smith, a former enslaved laborer born in 1859. The 1865 passage of the Thirteenth Amendment abolished slavery, and Smith and his family eventually purchased their property in Franklin County. He raised his children and grandchildren on that land. Claytor's grandfather repeatedly told her: "Do not hate. The heart has no room for hate. The heart works under the all or nothing principle. If you have a little drop of hate, it will come out."[17] She relied on his words often throughout her life.

Place as a construct is both the foundation and scaffold supporting and reinforcing personal identity. As Claytor negotiated aspects of segregation, she did so within a resurgent southern sectionalism that developed after World War II over divisive racial issues.[18] Claytor attended elementary and high school in the 1950s and 1960s during a time when the law supported segregation of schools, operating under the guise of "separate but equal." On May 17, 1954, the US Supreme Court affirmed *Brown v. Board of Education*, supporting education and equality advancement in the United States.[19]

Post the *Brown* decision, however, white Virginians grew increasingly wary of federal involvement in state affairs.[20] Organizers in Virginia countered the *Brown* ruling with militant political, social, and economic resistance, led by the Defenders of State Sovereignty and Individual Liberties.[21] Membership in this organization increased within its first year, with 30 chapters and 12,000 members in the state by the fall of 1955.[22] Supported by Virginia's Governor Thomas B. Stanley, the organization's influence reached far as it provided economic, social, and legal strategies for barring Virginia's implementation of racial integration.[23] Led by Senator Harry F. Byrd, Jr., a former governor, conservative lawmakers called upon the state to carry out systematic acts of massive resistance,[24] and Virginians literally closed their schools to prevent integration.[25] This act of resistance across the state further substantiated the unfixed position of place: the classroom symbolized federal rhetoric affirming black students' access to desegregated public schools while state sovereignty upheld black exclusion.

Virginia government leaders took advantage of the state constitution's Section 141 and denied funds to schools that complied with the *Brown* decision. On January 9, 1957, government leaders created addendums to support private school vouchers for white families, which provided an educational alternative for white children whose schools closed. The new option honored the Defenders of State Sovereignty and Individual Liberties' mission, to deny federally forced racial mixing and learning in public institutions.[26] The organization called upon all its members to act and remain vigilant, affirming:

> There will be no integration in Virginia only so long as the people are willing to stand unafraid and with a determination that is unfaltering. Part of this responsibility rests on your shoulders. Get busy, visit, call, telegraph, or write your representative and urge him to stand on your side, not on the side of the integrationist, NAACP, Virginia Council on Human Relations and others who are trying to force the evils of integration upon us. NOW IS THE TIME FOR ACTION![27]

Not all Virginians supported massive resistance. Along with the NAACP, the Virginia Council on Human Relations, a statewide organization of bi-racial members, organized to support school desegregation and other equal opportunity issues.[28] Still, Virginians elected Democrat Lindsay Almond, Jr., as governor in 1957, who promptly upheld former Governor Stanley's segregationist practices.[29] Following multiple state lawsuits, however, nine Virginia public schools received federal mandates to desegregate between 1957 and 1958.[30] At the same time, new allegiances developed across racial lines and counties to challenge school closings. On January 19, 1959, the US federal courts and Virginia courts ruled the state's school closings unconstitutional, leading Governor Almond to convene a special session with the General Assembly. He pledged his commitment to massive resistance, re-asserting publicly that Virginia "would not yield."[31] While his pledge drew from a false belief that Virginia's statehood took precedence over federal authority, he found that Virginia could not govern in isolation of federal laws.

Governor Almond eventually rescinded his pledge for massive resistance, yielding to federal and public pressure, despite his supporters' disapproval. Virginia passively tolerated desegregation, and the burden of actual enforcement remained with black students and their families. Massive resistance supporters continued fighting the strategy's dissolution. In September 1959, Prince Edward County shut down all its public schools in a final act of defiance. Public school closings affected black students' access to public education, while some white students entered private whites-only facilities.[32] It took Virginia half a decade before additional legislation influenced both the state's education and healthcare arenas.

Segregated Educational Experiences

Legislative changes in education and healthcare consistently met with staunch statewide opposition. The 1964 Civil Rights Act's Title VI ended sanctioned institutional segregation and discrimination in public spheres. Many predominately white and southern institutions continued to counter Title VI with active and passive defiance, leading the 1966 Medicare and Medicaid Certification Review Board to leverage financial accountability on Title VI non-compliant healthcare institutions. Failure to comply threatened their operational sustainability.[33]

New legislation gave black nurses and nursing students such as Claytor access to academic and clinical sectors formerly forbidden to them. While laws provided access, however, they did not guarantee protection.

As well, the newly-acquired registered nurse credential did not insulate them from racism and discrimination. Black nurses and nursing students were still black women in America, who navigated shifting geographical and social landscapes. As Darlene Clark Hine asserts, "The end of overt discrimination and segregation . . . did not mean the eradication of more subtle and sophisticated forms of institutionalized racism."[34] Researchers commend the resiliency of black nurses but rarely acknowledge the other side: that racism and exclusionary practices required black nurses to endure systematic weathering in their academic and professional pursuits.

To the Claytor family, the land held a sacredness, as a place of birth, sacrifice, celebration, and protection. The family land provided Claytor insulation from shame, countering negative representations by reinforcing the positive black identity. Indeed, black identity could be celebrated within the infrastructure of her home, the black community, and in the black classroom.

During massive resistance, Claytor's school in Franklin County, Virginia remained open and segregated for black students. She and her siblings attended Lee M. Waid, which encompassed grades one through twelve. The classroom provided significant buffering and equipping for navigating racialized discriminatory practices in Virginia through education. Black teachers created healing spaces of pride, safety, accountability, and possibilities for black students. Teachers replaced erroneous mainstream teachings of black inferiority with lessons that placed black men, women, and families at the center of their own worldview. Her love of learning and desire to escape home chores drove her school attendance. She found the classroom to be a welcomed break from canning, farming, and tending to her family's land.

Claytor admired and respected the black teachers at Lee M. Waid and considered teaching as a suitable career following graduation. This desire changed when her grandmother, Mary E. Smith, became ill. Claytor, a teenager, did not feel adequately equipped to manage her grandmother's care needs, yet she remained in the caregiver role. She was 16 years old when her grandmother died. Claytor sought a career in nursing, desiring never to feel that helpless again.[35]

After graduating from Lee M. Waid in 1961, Claytor relocated to the neighboring city of Roanoke, Virginia, where she and her sister, Lois Croan, attended the Burrell Memorial Hospital's Lucy Addison High School of Practical Nursing Program. For many women searching for nursing affiliations, vocational training programs were their only option.[36] Black physicians established Burrell Memorial Hospital in 1915 to serve the needs of black patients in the Roanoke area,[37] and its program provided formal education for many black nurses. It earned its accreditation in 1925 but later closed in 1934 during the Great Depression.[38] The nurse training program remained closed at Burrell Memorial Hospital for approximately 24 years.

On September 2, 1958, as massive resistance in Virginia was collapsing, Burrell Memorial Hospital partnered with the Roanoke City School System and established Lucy Addison High School of Practical Nursing. Claytor and her sister graduated from this school in 1963 as members of the first graduating class. Having received encouragement to further her educational pursuits, Claytor eventually attended Morgan State University, a historically black college in Baltimore, Maryland, where she took courses in general studies. She then enrolled in the Helene Fuld Provident Hospital's Registered Nursing Program located in Baltimore.[39]

Black physicians established Provident Hospital in 1894 with a twofold mission: to serve the healthcare needs of the black community and to provide an educational opportunity for black nurses and physicians.[40] Claytor excelled in her coursework and received recognition as "Miss Provident Hospital" in 1965. In historically black places such as Provident Hospital, black women could thrive in a context of mutual support and receive recognition for their accomplishments. Claytor gained valuable experience, confidence, and skills while attending the hospital's Registered Nursing Program. She graduated with a diploma in nursing in 1967 and continued to seek further opportunities to expand her role in the field of nursing while simultaneously working clinically to gain experience and earn a living.

In 1968, Claytor applied to and received acceptance into Roanoke College's School of Nursing program, following her aspiration to obtain a Bachelor of Science degree in Nursing. Once she received her acceptance letter, however, she discovered that the National League for Nursing (NLN) had not accredited the program. Claytor expressed to the academic office that she was seeking enrollment in an NLN-accredited program, knowing that, as a black woman, she had to continuously validate her education as one that was equal to her white counterparts. The institution's accreditation was more than an accolade; it was a means for upward mobility and resistance against racialized social hierarchies. In response, she applied to the NLN-accredited University of Virginia School of Nursing.[41]

Integrating the University of Virginia

The University of Virginia was among many public institutions wrestling, both internally and externally, with enforcing desegregation in the 1950s and 1960s. The University's School of Nursing remained without admittence of black students following the 1964 Civil Rights Act; but the fall semester of 1968 brought historic change. At that time, Roanoke College contacted the School of Nursing about a prospective transfer student, Claytor.

The first black student, a lawyer named Gregory Swanson of Martinsville, Virginia, enrolled in 1950 in the Law School's master's program. Admission occurred only after a prolonged court battle and the support of the NAACP's Legal Defense Fund.[42] Although he did not graduate, Swanson's admission paved the way for Walter Ridley to attend. Ridley became the first black student to graduate from the University of Virginia in 1953 with his Doctorate of Education.[43] What remains invisible in history are the other black students who were denied admission. Consequently, in a later interview, Swanson expressed: "Someday in the very near future the law school, as well as the whole university, will point the way to more constructive efforts in effectuating equality in the South. The University of Virginia should be the pivotal point of socio-economic and political changes which would make democracy a living reality."[44]

The University of Virginia Schools of Nursing and Education provided the only outlets for white women in the all-male student body. By the 1960s, more changes were coming. In 1961, the University admitted a black woman to the School of Education. Dean B.F.D. Runk wrote to the Assistant Dean of Women regarding Constance H (surname redacted on the record). He emphasized, "[S]he must be treated in accordance with the regular policies and procedures affecting all students and that denials of such applications can not [sic] be made on the basis of race."[45] At the same time, radical student protests gained attention at the University of Virginia, leading President Edgar Shannon to recognize the need for more open admissions policies. According to Historian Barbara Brodie, Dean Mary Lohr and other nursing faculty supported Shannon's decision to integrate. Yet the School of Nursing did not admit its first black student until 1968.[46]

That year, Claytor completed her transfer application for the University of Virginia's School of Nursing program. The application did not require an indication of race or ethnicity and the University accepted her for the fall enrollment, approximately 20 years after Swanson's arrival. Claytor grew up surrounded by the mountains in Franklin County, and as her family drove her into town, she found the mountains of Charlottesville to be a reminder of home. Her family said their goodbyes and dropped her off on the University's Grounds. After she arrived at McKim Hall, the nursing student dormitory, Claytor attempted registration for her assigned room. She immediately faced direct housing discrimination and isolation. The McKim Hall dormitory staff gave her a list of local hotel options under the auspices of no available space in the nursing dormitory.[47] Clearly, Dean Runk's 1961 prohibition of any denials "on the basis of race" was not heeded.

Claytor's family departed home, and the thought of leaving now was not an option. The NLN accredited the University of Virginia's nursing program, a requirement that Claytor firmly established before her admission. She traveled by foot, stopping at various hotels to inquire about obtaining a room. Although several hotels had vacancy signs in their windows to attract guests, upon her arrival the hotel employers all shared that they had no rooms. She continued walking and located another hotel that did accept her, and she stayed there for the initial weeks of the semester. She exhausted her savings, however, and could not personally sustain this unanticipated financial burden for more than a few weeks. Claytor then contacted the School of Nursing's Dean Lohr and submitted her formal resignation from the program. At that time, the Dean expressed her unawareness of the housing discrimination and expeditiously secured Claytor's room in McKim Hall, albeit in a segregated place.[48] Despite living in McKim, Claytor was not fully included in dormitory life as she never had a roommate for the duration of her education.

Claytor entered the bachelor's program with clinical experience and a well-rounded background, a strength that her peers and professors readily identified. She found the classroom and clinical setting to be a welcoming place, but this did not prevent or protect her against regular periods of loneliness and isolation. She often returned home to be with her family and attend church. As important places of acceptance, safety, and well-being, her home and church provided her with support and peace. She kept her bags packed in the dormitory, engaging the idea of remaining home during her weekend visits and not returning to the program. Claytor's mother would gently nudge her daughter, saying, "Wait another week; stay another week." Her mother regularly covered her in prayer with the reminder that she was capable of finishing.[49]

Claytor graduated in 1970 as the first black nurse to be admitted to and graduate from the University of Virginia School of Nursing. She returned to the historically black Burrell Memorial Hospital in Roanoke, Virginia, where she worked as a registered nurse on the general medical–surgical floor. Claytor also worked as a public health nurse. In 1976, she joined the US Department of Veterans Affairs Medical Center in Salem, Virginia, as a mental health nurse. Claytor's desire to pursue a second degree in nursing grew with continued exposure of new ideas and opportunities. She applied to the University of Virginia's School of Nursing program in 1983, and once again gained admission—this time into the master's program in mental health. She graduated in 1985 and continued working at Salem's Veterans Affairs Medical Center. After 30 years of dedicated and awarded service, Claytor retired as Service Line Chief Nurse for Geriatrics and Extended Care. On April 7, 2017, School of Nursing Dean Dorrie Fontaine offered a formal apology to Claytor, leading the way for one of the first formal apologies offered on behalf of the University of Virginia. It was an acknowledgment of the discriminatory practices that excluded black students from attending or fully engaging in University enrollment, matriculation, traditions, and student activities. The apology did not correct nor mitigate the past but instead illuminated it, serving as an acknowledgment of the institution's history.

Conclusion

Claytor and other black students in Virginia grew up during a time when the state led the South's defiance to racial equality. State leaders fought school desegregation until the federal courts intervened. Consequently, massive resistance delayed desegregation for over a decade, directly influencing and threatening black Virginian students' public-school access in areas such as Charlottesville, Front Royal, New Kent, Norfolk, and Prince Edward County Schools.[50] In this context, Claytor navigated both segregated and integrated places throughout her educational journey. Her case study illustrates the convergence of historical yet evolving places with socio-political changes in the lived experience of one black woman in Virginia.

Researchers commend the resiliency of black nurses—that they were able to overcome "life on the margins" of an oppressive racial system. However, were they resilient to the effects of these experiences? Researchers rarely acknowledge the other side: that racism and exclusionary practices required black nurses to endure real and anticipated dangers at the expense of desegregating spaces. Place was never "fixed" for them.[51] Still, as they navigated these moving lines, black nurses were central figures in the integration of the US healthcare system. As black women pursued their academic, professional, and personal goals, they traversed a tenuous path to institutional integration, while simultaneously shouldering the compounding burdens of race, gender, and class. Black nurses and nursing students elected to enter newly desegregated spaces, often aware of the unequal demands yet still choosing to pursue advancement in the nursing field. Their narratives elucidate how place shapes, informs, and complicates both personal and group mobility.

Notes

1. Aspects of this article come from an interview by the author with Mavis Claytor during the McGehee Lecture, "A Conversation with Mavis Claytor (MSN '85, BSN '70)," April 10, 2017, at the University of Virginia School of Nursing. A recording of this interview can be accessed at https://www.nursing.virginia.edu/alumni/get-connected/mcgehee/. The Institutional Review Board at the University of Virginia approved the study, and additional interviews have taken place.

2. Kevin R. Hardwick and Warren R. Hofstra, *Virginia Reconsidered: New Histories of the Old Dominion* (Charlottesville: University of Virginia Press, 2003); and Maurie D. McInnis, *To Be Sold: Virginia and the American Slave Trade Exhibit, The Interstate Slave Trade* (Richmond: Library of Virginia, 2014), accessed May 10, 2018, http://www.virginiamemory.com/online-exhibitions/exhibits/show/to-be-sold/the-interstate-slave-trade.

3. McInnis, *To Be Sold*, website, sections in "Introduction," and "Robert Lumpkin."

4. Fraser D. Neiman, "The Lost World of Monticello: An Evolutionary Perspective," *Journal of Anthropological Research* 64, no. 2 (2008): 161–93. See also "Property: How Many People Did Thomas Jefferson Own?" According to *The Jefferson Monticello*, "Thomas Jefferson enslaved over 600 human beings throughout the course of his life. 400 people were enslaved at Monticello; the other 200 people were held in bondage on Jefferson's other properties. At any given time, around 130 people were enslaved at Monticello." See *The Jefferson Monticello*, Charlottesville, Virginia, accessed December 20, 2018, https://www.monticello.org/site/plantation-and-slavery/property.

5. Thomas Jefferson, "Excerpt: Query XIV, The Administration of Justice and Description of the Laws?" *Notes on the State of Virginia*, accessed July 26, 2018, http://xroads.virginia.edu//jefferson/ch14.html.

6. Correspondence from Edna M. Lee, R.N., to Miss Margaret E. Gray, Educational Director Virginia State Board of Examiners, November 16, 1967, MS-8, Brodie Box 1, Folder 10, Eleanor Crowder Bjoring Center for Nursing Historical Inquiry; "Dixie Hospital," Historical Collections & Services, Claude Moore Health Sciences Library, Charlottesville, Virginia. See also "Roanoke News," in *Richmond Planet* 39, no. 29 (Richmond, Virginia: May 27, 1922), 8; and correspondence from Mabel E. Montgomery, R.N., M.A., Secretary-Treasurer, to Miss Etuy E. Hall, R.N., Director, Piedmont Sanatorium, October 7, 1966, in RG 37, Department of Health Professions Board of Nursing 1947–1979, Box 1, AC 35095, Piedmont Sanatorium, Library of Virginia, Richmond, Virginia.

7. Katherine McKittrick, *Demonic Grounds: Black Women and the Cartographies of Struggle* (Minneapolis: University of Minnesota Press, 2006); and LaKisha Michelle Simmons, *Crescent City Girls: The Lives of Young Black Women in Segregated New Orleans* (Chapel Hill: The University of North Carolina Press, 2015).

8. McKittrick, "Demonic Grounds," 143.

9. Simmons, *Crescent City Girls*, 28.

10. Sharla Fett, *Working Cures: Healing, Health, and Power on Southern Slave Plantations* (Chapel Hill: University of North Carolina Press, 2002); Darlene Clark Hine, *Black Women in White: Racial Conflict and Cooperation in the Nursing Profession, 1890–1950* (Bloomington: Indiana University Press, 1989), 3–25.

11. Georgia Burnette, "Black Nurses Struggle for Admission to Professional Schools: Four Retired Nurses Look Back," *Reflections 10, no. 1* (2004): 65–72. https://reflectionsnarrativesofprofessionalhelp

12. Josepha Campinha-Bacote, "The Black Nurses' Struggle toward Equality: An Historical Account of the National Association of Colored Graduate Nurses," *Journal of National Black Nurses Association* 2, no. 2 (1988): 15–25.

13. Leslie A. Falk, "The Negro American's Health and the Medical Committee for Human Rights," *Medical Care* 4, no. 3 (1966): 171–77; Lottie Ozias Harris, "Where Is the Black Nurse?" *American Journal of Nursing* 72, no. 2 (February 1972): 282–84; David Barton Smith, "Population Ecology and the Racial Integration of Hospitals and Nursing Homes in the United States," *Milbank Quarterly* 68, no. 4 (1990): 571–75; Jill Quadagno, "Promoting Civil Rights through the Welfare State: How Medicare Integrated Southern Hospitals," *Social Problems* 47, no. 1 (2000): 223–44; and Karen Kruse Thomas, "Dr. Jim Crow: The University of North Carolina, the Regional Medical School for Negroes, and the Desegregation of Southern Medical Education, 1945–1960," *Journal of African American History* 88, no. 3, 223–44.

14. Falk, "The Negro American's Health," 172–74; See also Khalil Gibran Muhamad, *The Condemnation of Blackness: Race, Crime, and the Making of Modern Urban America* Cambridge, MA: Harvard University Press, 2011); and *Plessy vs. Ferguson*, Judgment, Decided May 18, 1896; Records of the Supreme Court of the United States; Record Group 267; *Plessy v. Ferguson*, 163, #15248, National Archives, accessed May 10, 2018, http://www.ourdocuments.gov/doc.php?flash=true&doc=52.

15. Falk, "The Negro American's Health," 172.

16. U.S. Department of Health, Education and Welfare, *Vital Statistics of the United States*, vol. 1 (Washington, DC: United States Government Printing Office, 1950), 1–31.

17. Wyatt Smith quote obtained from interview with Mavis Claytor, McGehee Lecture.

18. Dewey W. Grantham, *The South in Modern America: A Region at Odds* (New York: Harper, 2001).

19. Quadagno, "Promoting Civil Rights through the Welfare State," 74–77; and "No. 1. Appeal from The United States District Court for The District of Kansas," *Brown et al. v. Board of Education of Topeka et al.*, October Term 1953: 483–91, Princeton University Harvey S. Firestone Memorial Library, Princeton, New Jersey, accessed May 10, 2018, https://www.princeton.edu//Brown1.pdf. See also C. Vann Woodward, *The Strange Career of Jim Crow* (New York: Oxford University Press, 1974).

20. J. Douglas Smith, *Managing White Supremacy, Race, Politics, and Citizenship in Jim Crow Virginia* (Chapel Hill & London: The University of North Carolina Press, 2002), 9.

21. David Pembroke Neff, "The Defenders of State Sovereignty and Individual Liberties," *Encyclopedia Virginia*, Virginia Foundation for the Humanities, 2013, accessed May 10, 2018, https://www.encyclopediavirginia.org/Defenders_of_State_Sovereignty_and_Individual_Liberties; Frank B. Atkinson, *The Dynamic Dominion, Revised Second Edition: Realignment and the Rise of Two-Party Competition in Virginia, 1945–1980* (Lanham: Rowman & Littlefield Publishers, Inc, 2007), 83–98; and "Correspondence from Defenders of State Sovereignty and Individual Liberties Special Bulletin to Our Membership," 1956, in Organizational Records 1956–1963, Folder, BC 0007431295, AC 39469, Library of Virginia, Richmond, Virginia.

22. Neff, "The Defenders of State Sovereignty and Individual Liberties."

23. "Correspondence from Defenders of State Sovereignty," 1–3. See also William B. Foster, Jr., "Gray to Head on Barring Integration: Stanley Says Find Legal Way," *Richmond News Leader*, September 13, 1954 (n.p), Valentine Museum, Richmond, Virginia.

24. James H. Hershman, Jr., "Massive Resistance," *Encyclopedia Virginia*, Virginia Foundation for the Humanities, 2011, accessed May 10, 2018, https://www.encyclopediavirginia.org/Massive_Resistance. See also Neff, "The Defenders of State Sovereignty and Individual Liberties;" Atkinson, *The Dynamic Dominion*, 83–87; and "Correspondence from Defenders of State Sovereignty," 1–3.

25. Neff, "The Defenders of State Sovereignty and Individual Liberties."

26. Atkinson, *The Dynamic Dominion*, 95–98; Hershman, "Massive Resistance."

27. "Correspondence from Defenders of State Sovereignty," 3.

28. "College of William and Mary Virginia Council on Human Relations," *William and Mary Libraries*, accessed July 26, 2018, https://libraries.wm.edu/exhibits/virginia-council-human-relations.

29. Atkinson, *The Dynamic Dominion*, 99–112 and 115–19; and Hershman, "Massive Resistance."

30. Hershman, "Massive Resistance."

31. Hershman, "Massive Resistance"; Atkinson, "The Dynamic Dominion," 116–17.

32. Hershman, "Massive Resistance"; Atkinson, *The Dynamic Dominion*, 116–23.

33. David Barton Smith, "Population Ecology and the Racial Integration of Hospitals and Nursing Homes in the United States," *Milbank Quarterly* 68, no. 4 (1990): 823–70. See also Quadagno, "Promoting Civil Rights through the Welfare State."

34. Hine, *Black Women in White*, 191.

35. McGehee Lecture.

36. Phoebe Ann Pollitt, *African American and Cherokee Nurses in Appalachia: A History, 1900–1965* (Jefferson: McFarland and Company, 2016), 154.

37. National Register of Historic Places Registration Form, "Burrell Memorial Hospital," OMB No. 1024-0018 (Submission date: 2003). See also John Davis, "Black Roanoke: Our Story," February 3, 2014, accessed May 10, 2018, https://www.roanokeva.gov/DocumentCenter/View/1537/Black-Roanoke-Our-Story?bidId=.

38. National Register of Historic Places Registration Form, "Burrell Memorial Hospital."

39. McGehee Lecture.

40. Robert L. Jackson and Emerson C. Walden, "A History of Provident Hospital, Baltimore, Maryland," *Journal of National Medical Associations* 59, no. 3 (1967): 157–65. For a history of the Black hospital movement, see Vanessa Northington Gamble, *Making a Place for Ourselves: The Black Hospital Movement, 1920–1945* (New York: Oxford University Press, 1995).

41. McGehee Lecture.

42. "Martinsville Negro Lawyer Is Admitted to University," *Richmond Times-Dispatch*, September 16, 1950; and "U.Va. Faces Suit for Rejection of Negro as Law School Student," *Richmond Times-Dispatch*, July 26, 1950. "Gregory H. Swanson: First African American Admitted to U.Va." (1950), from the

William R. Kenan Jr. Endowment Fund for the Academic Village of the University of Virginia, Charlottesville, Virginia, accessed December 10, 2015, http://www.virginia.edu/woodson/projects/kenan/swanson/swanson.html.

43. "U.Va. Enrolls Negro, Ph.D. Candidate," *Richmond News Leader*, September 27, 1950, from the William R. Kenan Jr. Endowment Fund for the Academic Village of the University of Virginia, accessed December 10, 2015, http://www.virginia.edu/woodson/projects/kenan/swanson/nl92750enrolls.jpg. See also "The Life of Walter N. Ridley," Ridley Scholarship Fund, Ridley at The University of Virginia, accessed December 16, 2018, https://aig.alumni.virginia.edu/ridley/about/history/life-walter-n-ridley/.

44. "First Negro Student Gives Views on U.Va." Unprocessed News Clipping, University in Virginia's Alderman Library Collection, University of Virginia, Charlottesville, Virginia.

45. "Letter, B.F.D. Runk to Mrs. Charles W. McNitt," July 28, 1961, University of Virginia Special Collections, accessed July 26, 2018, https://explore.lib.virginia.edu/exhibits/show/uvawomen/breakingtradition.

46. Barbara Brodie, *Mr. Jefferson's Nurses: University of Virginia School of Nursing, 1901–2001* (Charlottesville: Rector and Visitors of the University of Virginia, 2000).

47. McGehee Lecture.

48. Ibid.

49. Ibid.

50. Hershman, "Massive Resistance."

51. Simmons, *Crescent City Girls*, 28.

Disclosure. The author has no relevant financial interest or affiliations with any commercial interests related to the subjects discussed within this article.

VICTORIA TUCKER, RN, BSN, PhD(c)
University of Virginia School of Nursing
The Eleanor Crowder Bjoring Center for Nursing Historical Inquiry
McLeod Hall
202 Jeanette Lancaster Way
Charlottesville, VA 22903

Filipino Nurses and the US Navy at Hampton Roads, Virginia: The Importance of Place

Reynaldo Capucao Jr.
University of Virginia

"Place" has great relevance for understanding the workings of Filipino nurses at specific times in history. Following the arguments of J. Nicholas Entrikin, this article shows how "human experience is always rooted in place."[1] In particular, it examines Filipino nurses in the United States as a reflection of their locations in proximity to American naval bases such as the Hampton Roads region in Virginia. Filipino-Americans, an understudied immigrant group, have had a substantial impact on the nursing profession in Virginia, nationally, and internationally. Indeed, in the United States, Filipino nurses constitute a crucial labor supply, comprising the majority of internationally educated nurses in the country. Because Naval Station Norfolk, the largest naval base in the world with the largest Filipino population on the East coast, resides within Hampton Roads, this area became a place for the migration of Filipino nurses. It influenced their futures, and that of nursing, in significant ways. Indeed, the vibrancy of Naval Station Norfolk in Hampton Roads, Virginia, as a site for Filipino nursing cultivation illuminates the centrality of place for Filipino nurses.

The concept of "place" also has relevance for understanding the workings of imperialism. Indeed, race, gender, class, and culture were important in shaping Filipino nurses' experiences in the United States. The professional education of Filipino nurses dates back to the late nineteenth and early twentieth centuries after the United States defeated Spain in the Spanish American War. This was a formative time for United States overseas expansion. The military played an important role during the war as an outlet for white nurses, who had worked during the war, to gain permanent professional recognition back home. Then newly professionalized American nurses came to the Philippines and forged a modern nursing identity among Filipino nurses based on

Nursing History Review 28 (2020): 158–169. A Publication of the American Association for the History of Nursing. Copyright © 2020 Springer Publishing Company.
http://dx.doi.org/10.1891/1062-8061.28.158

the American model, creating what Catherine Ceniza Choy calls an "empire of care."[2] A half century later, the first mass migration of Filipino nurses occurred during the 1950s, and as of 2017, out of 2,906,840 active registered nurses employed in the United States, it is estimated that 200,000 are of Philippine origin—approximately 7% of the total nursing workforce.[3] Most studies on Filipino nurses either sort them under the Asian umbrella category, emphasize professional migration through economic logic, or portray them as statistical numbers. As Choy argues, however, this renders Filipino nurses as "impersonal, faceless objects of study, an objectification that prevents an understanding and appreciation of these migrants as multidimensional historical agents, and consequently hinders an identification with them as professionals, women, and immigrants."[4] Despite Filipino-Americans forming a sizable portion of the state's nursing workforce, the Virginia Department of Health Professions' publication, "Virginia's Registered Nurse Workforce: 2017," does not distinguish Filipino nurses from other Asian nurses.[5] This article uses Hampton Roads as a site to recognize a wider history of Filipino nurses.

Hampton Roads and Naval Station Norfolk as a Location for Filipino Immigration

The Hampton Roads area is often called "America's First Region" due to Jamestown's establishment in 1607. Prior to the establishment of a naval base, this region surrounding the Chesapeake Bay had already proven to be of great significance in US naval history. The Revolutionary War reached its end with the 1781 Battle of the Chesapeake, ensuring America's victory with French naval ships blockading British forces at Yorktown. During the Civil War, the Confederate Army built defenses at Sewell's Point, the future site of Naval Station Norfolk, to control Virginia's Tidewater region. Offshore in 1862, the *Monitor* and the *Merrimack* fought in the Battle of Hampton Roads—the first battle in history between ironclad ships.

In 1907, the Jamestown Exposition at Sewell's Point celebrated the 300th anniversary of the Jamestown colony, and it also supported the idea of a federal naval base. With the onset of the First World War in 1917, under President Woodrow Wilson's discretion, a naval base was constructed in Norfolk, Virginia. By 1939, extensive funding resulted in the naval base being the largest of all the Navy's training stations. As the Second World War got underway, on July 19, 1940, Congress instituted the "two-ocean Navy," which accelerated defense production and expanded the naval base with machines and ships to be used as a supply depot for Allied Forces.[6] The need for labor led naval officials to recruit more men to build 11 new barracks, a dining hall, and attendant auxiliary facilities.[7] It became Naval Station Norfolk at Hampton Roads. The base's expansion was crucial in 1941 after the attack on Pearl Harbor, which pushed the United States' entrance into the war. At that time, Pearl Harbor was the largest American naval base in the Pacific Ocean, and the attack meant further government reliance on other naval bases. Since then, Norfolk's naval base has continued to expand and shape the surrounding area into the twenty-first century.[8]

Naval bases in the United States were especially important in enveloping Filipino nurses because of immigration policies that favored filial relationships. These forces are illuminated in a case study of Hampton Roads' Naval Station Norfolk. After the Spanish American War, the United States established a naval station in the Philippines at Subic Bay in 1901, which became its largest overseas base.[9] US naval connections continued after the National Origins Act of 1924, which restricted immigration from many nations based on quotas. It did not, however, apply to protectorates of the United States, such as the Philippines, and a wave of Filipino immigration occurred. The US Navy reinforced American imperial objectives by recruiting Filipino men in non-combative roles initially as mess attendants and stewards. As one source notes, "Filipinos were the only foreign nationals allowed to enlist in the U.S. armed forces without first immigrating to this country. And the Navy was the only military branch they could join."[10] The Nationality Act of 1940 enabled foreign service men serving at least 3 years in the armed forces to be naturalized as American citizens. The Second World War and its aftermath drastically increased Filipino service men in the US Navy. Gradually, the recruitment process expanded into combat roles upon the Philippines' political independence in 1946. Between 1944 and 1946, 2,200 Filipino men enlisted in the US Navy. As well, in 1946, the War Brides Act allowed Filipino service men's spouses and children to enter the United States as non-quota immigrants.[11] The passage of the Military Bases Agreement in 1947 formalized continued military cooperation between the United States and the newly independent Philippines by allowing the enlistment of Filipino citizens into the US Navy.[12] From 1953 to 1958, the number of Filipino service men doubled to 5,525.[13] By 1976, approximately 17,000 Filipinos served in the Navy.[14] Despite the Agreement expiring in 1992, thousands of Filipinos had already enlisted as service men and attained American citizenship, with a large settlement of Filipino communities around naval stations.

Filipino-American Nurses in Hampton Roads

As noted earlier, the expansion of Filipino nursing dates back to the late nine-teenth and early twentieth centuries. Several authors have written about the influence of American nurses on Filipino women at this time.[15] Indeed, the importation of an Americanized version of nursing inevitably prepared Fil-ipino nurses toward American healthcare instead of focusing on the welfare of the Philippines. In 1907, the US government established the Philippine General Hospital School of Nursing as the first government-funded train-ing school. Similar to their American counterparts, Filipino nurses used the nursing profession as a vehicle to create opportunities for socioeconomic advancement. The nurse's white cap, important as an Americanization symbol, became symbolic of status for Filipino nurses.[16] As early as 1911, philanthropic institutions like the Rockefeller Foundation, the Daughters of the American Revolution, and the Catholic Scholarship Fund sponsored Filipino nurses to further their training in the United States with the expectation that they would return to the Philippines to propagate modern nursing knowledge they had ascertained. The social exchange piqued Filipino nurses' newfound indepen-dence and created a glimpse of the world beyond the Islands.[17]

Although important to Filipino nurses' history in the United States, a focus on imperialism alone denies the importance of "place" as a site for resistance—where Filipino nurses could imagine new lives for themselves. Nursing provided the ability for Filipino women to be independent and explore the world. Beginning in the early twentieth century, financial support from private institutions sponsoring Filipino nurses' education in the United States was the primary route out of the country for them. This changed after the Second World War, as the United States faced a critical nursing short-age with the expansion of hospitals, increased acuity of patients, and higher insurance coverage of American citizens. Concurrently, the Philippines had an overabundance of nurses and suffered from high rates of nurse unemployment. The intersectionality of these events together with American nursing recruit-ment policies created the perfect environment for the eventual migration of Filipino nurses.[18]

Barbara Brush has written about foreign nurse immigrants to American hospitals. She notes that in 1950, the Rockefeller Foundation commissioned American nurse consultant Lorena Murray to determine the Philippine's ability for "self-containment in the production of nurses" by examining nurse teaching facilities and measuring nurse production rates. Her survey team reported that the country had the "right kind of nursing leadership," but was concerned with the "right type" of nurse to care for the country's needs.[19] Despite an overabundance of professional nurses trained in the American model of nursing, Filipino nurses were unprepared to handle the vast health disparities between urban and rural populations. Therefore, their professional skillset did not fit into the agrarian economy of their home country, which could only employ a marginal number of nurses; this led many Filipino nurses to seek alternative means of employment.[20]

The mass migration of Filipino nurses began in 1951 with the Exchange Visitor Program (EVP). This coincided with the growth of hospitals, with Hill-Burton funding, that created a greater need for nurses. By the late 1960's, Filipinos constituted the majority of EVP exchanges. By 1973, more than 12,000 Filipino nurses had entered the United States through the EVP.[21] This wave of migration was also marked by the passage of the Naturalization and Immigration Act of 1965, which exponentially increased the visibility of Filipino nurses. This Act favored the immigration of Filipino nurses by abolishing the national origins quota system. It also implemented a preference procedure that allowed immigrants who possessed education, skills, and filial relationships to citizens to come to the United States. In 1970, the United States amended the temporary status of occupational H-1 visas to enable permanent employment and accommodate the needs of hospitals. This afforded Filipino nurses more opportunities for American citizenship and the ability to avoid the EVP's mandatory clause of returning to their country of origin after 2 years. Between 1965 and 1972, Filipino nurses employed in American hospitals increased 400%.[22]

During the mid-twentieth century, Filipino nurses became a pipeline to fill nurse shortages around the world with nursing schools rapidly proliferating to accommodate a steady stream of nurses. In 1970, World Health Organization nurse consultant Helen Mussalem surveyed Philippine nursing schools and curricula and noted that they reflected the needs of industrialized countries.[23] The migration was also exacerbated by the Philippine government's desire to increase the country's gross domestic product through overseas worker remittances. This is viewable through Philippine President Ferdinand Marcos' 1973 address to the Philippine Nurses Association:

> We intend to take care of [Filipino nurses] but as we encourage this migration, I repeat, we will now encourage the training of all nurses because as I repeat, this is a market that we should take advantage of. Instead of stopping the nurses from going abroad why don't we produce more nurses? If they want one thousand nurses we produce a thousand more.[24]

A lack of job opportunity and monetary support from the Philippines and the ability to apply for American citizenship without requiring employment by a hospital fueled the diaspora of Filipino nurses across the United States. Chain migration was influential. Filipino nurses followed other Filipinos to particular destinations, including the naval base at Hampton Roads, Virginia.

Hampton Roads became a place for Filipino newlyweds to settle. This region depicts a distinct migration pattern separate from historically concentrated areas of foreign-trained nurses, specifically at inner-city hospitals in New York, Michigan, New Jersey, California, and Illinois. The significant naval presence in Hampton Roads, which had cultivated a respectable number of Filipino service men, also attracted other Filipino migrants, thereby fostering the largest Filipino community on the East Coast.[25] For example, the pioneering Filipino nurses who settled in Hampton Roads often arrived through marriage with a Filipino service man. As households of Filipino nurses and service men increased, the Filipino community continued to grow by attracting relatives and friends to the area, which included more nurses.[26] Thus, Filipino service men stationed at the naval base significantly influenced the migration patterns of Filipino nurses.

The central tenet of family in Filipino culture reinforced the importance of settling down, getting married, and establishing a community. There have been accounts of Filipino sailors stationed in Norfolk filling two Greyhound buses, traveling to Philadelphia for weekend trips, and lining hospital sidewalks where many Filipino nurses worked. Some would then continue to Atlantic City for entertainment and courtship. Marriage would lead Filipino nurses to Hampton Roads, despite that not being their initial destination. Rebecca Tolentino was one of the nurses in Philadelphia courted by a sailor. She followed her husband, who was stationed in Annapolis, Maryland, before finally being commissioned to Naval Station Norfolk. Some Filipino nurses could not handle the constant moving. Liz Ligana, whose husband worked in a submarine, moved from Maine, to Mississippi, to Connecticut, to Pennsylvania, and finally to Virginia, where she told her husband, "No more, I'm not moving!"[27] Other Filipino nurses, like Jessica Bello, married their husbands in the Philippines and followed them to Naval Station Norfolk at Hampton Roads.[28]

A small minority of women nurses married Filipino sailors to acquire citizenship so that they could continue their service to American hospitals, maintain their newfound independence, and avoid the temporary status of the EVP and occupational visas. Regardless of the reason for residency in Hampton Roads, the union between Filipino nurses and naval service men created the foundation for one of the most concentrated Filipino-American communities in the country. Despite the end of the Military Bases Agreement, chain migration has continually expanded the Filipino-American population and number of Filipino service men, nurses, and nursing ancillary staff in Hampton Roads and other naval areas.

A Sense of Place

The naval base at Hampton Roads is not only a physical locality but also can be seen as fostering a "sense of place," a cultural space where social conflict occurred. Although the US Navy is known for its diversity and supported a culturally heterogeneous Hampton Roads, pioneering Filipino nurses still faced discrimination as they arrived during the country's transition toward racial equality. Officially, the Navy desegregated in 1946 and the American Nurses Association (ANA) in 1950; yet neither was immune to the racial attitudes of the time.[29] For instance, at the height of Filipino nurse migration, in 1968, Doris De Vincenzo, the Director of the ANA's International Program, advised state nurses associations and state boards of nursing of the potential complications caused by the increasing foreign-trained nurse labor force. She warned that "it will mean continuing problems in establishing high school and nursing preparation for licensure, in acquiring English language fluency, and in becoming oriented to the complexities of our healthcare system."[30]

De Vincenzo's statement reflected the discriminatory behaviors faced by Filipino nurses in Hampton Roads. When attempting to move up the clinical ladder or receive post-graduate education, they often faced resistance from hospitals. However, these nurses handled deterrents differently. Despite being a qualified candidate, Rebecca Tolentino, one of the first Filipino nurses who applied to Norfolk General Hospital's School of Anesthesia, recollected the program director dissuading her application. Disregarding this pushback, Tolentino fought for her acceptance into the 1971 class and was successfully admitted. In another example, Nita Cacanindin was recently promoted to head nurse, and despite her newfound authority and responsibility, she experienced discrimination when hospital staff were unwilling to learn the correct pronunciation of her last name. Tired of facing harassment, she ignored a page when she was addressed as "Mrs. Caca Indian"; later, the person who paged her asked why she did not answer, and she said, ". . . because you called me different. That is not my name."[31] By contrast, Loreto Montano dealt with prejudicial scheduling by focusing on proving her proficiency as a nurse, until eventually she gained fellow co-workers' friendship and more desirable shifts.[32]

Clarita Miraflor's 1976 study examined Filipino nurses' experiences in Chicago metropolitan hospitals, with 60% of her participants identifying as having exchange visitor visas.[33] Thus, most of her participants were employed in staff nurse positions before arrival in the United States. A majority of her participants stated that they identified better with white nurses compared to black nurses, and non-white ancillary nursing staff resisted their authority. This contrasts with the more positive experiences between Filipino and African American nursing staff in Hampton Roads. Many Filipino nurses who arrived to this region were unemployed upon entry into the United States, so they simultaneously worked as nurse's aides and studied to take the National Council Licensure Examination (NCLEX) to become registered nurses. For example, arriving in 1986, Jolly Capucao worked as a nurse's aide at Beth Sholom Village, a nursing home in Virginia Beach, alongside other unlicensed Filipino nurses. Together, they studied for the NCLEX and took the exam in Baltimore, Maryland, instead of Virginia, due to the less stringent licensure requirements for foreign-trained nurses. Despite failing the exam three times, Capucao became the first among her group to obtain her state licensure for nursing in 1990.[34] Additionally, because Filipino nurse migrants in Hampton Roads usually began as nurse's aides, they tended to work more closely with other underrepresented groups such as African Americans. This created a sense of collegiality between nursing staff of color in Hampton Roads as they worked up the clinical ladder together. Thus, as white women set up a hierarchy of nursing that segregated African Americans, a different set of relationships developed in Hampton Roads. Filipino nurses' experiences with African Americans provide new insights to the conflicts and ties that bind nurses of different races and ethnicities together.

At the same time, "place" became more tightly bound for Filipinos as they created separate enclaves for themselves. Hampton Roads also became a site for community support for nurses. To overcome racist attitudes of the time, Filipino nurses not only created a sense of community with nurses of color in the workplace, but they also formed a Filipino nursing community. In 1978, the Philippine Nurses Association of Tidewater, or PNAT, currently known as the Philippine Nurses Association of Virginia, was founded to connect Filipino nurses in the area and provide personal and professional growth to Filipino nurses in Virginia.[35] The organization's objectives included assisting nurses to pass the NCLEX, providing a voice for Filipino nurses, and creating a sense of community. The PNAT also provided classes in English to help Filipino nurses struggling to find jobs due to Virginia's reticence to hire foreign-trained nurses because of the presumed language barrier. The PNAT worked alongside the Council of United Filipino Organizations of Tidewater, a conglomeration of Filipino organizations in Hampton Roads, to build a stronger sense of community. In 2000, the Council built the Philippine Cultural Center of Virginia, the largest Filipino cultural center in the United States at the time.[36] The formation of the PNAT provided a platform for Filipino nurses' voices within Virginia's nursing community, as several members, such as Perry Francisco and Levy Paler, previously served on Virginia's State Board of Nursing. Thus, to be Filipino in these places was a privilege.

There is a downside to this story of place. A growing number of Filipino nurses migrating to Hampton Roads were unprepared to handle work in the American healthcare system, which resulted from receiving an inadequate education from newer and less reputable schools back home. The ongoing influx of Filipino nurses into Hampton Roads over the decades reflected the commodification and commercialization of people in the Philippines and the deterioration of quality Filipino nurses. President Marcos' plan encouraged this commodification and the rapid proliferation of nursing schools in the Philippines over the next decades.

In 1996, the PNAT's first president, Araceli Marcial, created the Abbott Education Center, a certified nurse's aide program, in Virginia Beach. This Center helped to acculturate foreign-educated health professionals to the United States. Marcial had arrived in 1960 through the EVP at Newark, New Jersey, before settling in Hampton Roads with her naval husband in 1970. After more than 60 years of nursing experience shared between the Philippines and the United States, Marcial, now 82-years-old, continues to further nursing's professionalization by working as the Abbott Education Center's program director and teaching any student interested in practicing nursing. She also encourages Filipino nurse migrants to sit for the NCLEX and move beyond the baccalaureate degree. However, she has noticed that many incoming Filipino nurse migrants are unwilling or unprepared to take the exam. The attitudes of the newer generation of Filipino nurse migrants are understandable, as they receive higher salaries as American nurse's aides than they would as nurses in the Philippines, and they have greater job opportunities. In addition, these new nurse migrants have the support of family and community in Hampton Roads that was unfamiliar to their original counterparts.[37]

Conclusion

The direct link between American naval assignments and international and domestic migration patterns influenced the spread of Filipino nursing to Hampton Roads. With roots in the Spanish American War, the naval bases it created and the growth of Filipino nursing along the American model emerged within an imperialist context. Filipino men filled the ranks of the US Navy, and Filipino nurses implemented an American model of professional nursing. Thus, this localized history of Filipino nurses in Hampton Roads provides greater comprehension of the noteworthy relationship between the professionalization of nursing, military affairs, migration, and places where these forces intersect. The large Filipino community at Hampton Roads is attributable to naval service men and their brides, the need for healthcare professionals, and chain migration of Filipino citizens' family members. At the same time, Filipino nurses' experiences fit into the larger historical narrative of women using the nursing profession as a vehicle for socioeconomic mobility. The intersectionality of events in the global arena together with American nursing and naval recruitment policies at the local level created a key place for the diaspora of Filipino nurses around naval stations in the United States.

Notes

1. J. Nicholas Entrikin, "Place, Region, and Modernity," in *The Power of Place: Bringing Together Geographical and Sociological Imaginations*, eds. John A. Agnew and James S. Duncan (New York: Routledge, 1989), 30–43. Quotation is on p. 41.

2. Catherine Ceniza Choy, *Empire of Care: Nursing and Migration in Filipino American History* (Durham: Duke University Press, 2003); See also Yen Le Espiritu, *Home Bound: Filipino American Lives across Cultures, Communities, and Countries* (Berkeley: University of California Press, 2003); and Dorothy B. Fujita-Rony, *American Workers, Colonial Power: Philippine Seattle and the Transpacific West, 1919–1941* (Berkeley: University of California Press, 2003).

3. Bureau of Labor Statistics, "Occupational Employment and Wages, May 2017: 29–1141 Registered Nurses," *Occupational Employment Statistics,* May 2017, updated March 30, 2018, https://www.bls.gov/Oes/current/oes291141.htm. Accessed May 29, 2018; See also Danny Tex Van M. Ardenio, "Why Filipino Nurses Work Abroad," *Panay News,* January 16, 2018, https://www.pressreader.com/philippines/panay-news/20180116/281586651004151. Accessed May 30, 2018.

4. Choy, *Empire of Care,* 3.

5. Healthcare Workforce Data Center, ed., "Virginia's Registered Nurse Workforce: 2017," (October 2017): 6, (http://www.dhp.virginia.gov/media/dhpweb/docs/hwdc/nurse/0001RN2017.pdf). Accessed on May 29, 2018.

6. Hampton Roads Naval Historical Foundation, ed., *Images of America: Naval Station Norfolk* (Charleston: Arcadia Publishing, 2014), 8.

7. Ibid.

8. Old Dominion University Regional Studies Institute, ed., "The Filipino American Community," (2007) in *State of the Region Reports: Hampton Roads. 101.* (September 2007), 49–61. https://digitalcommons.odu.edu/sor_reports/101. Accessed on May 29, 2018.

9. Ben Barber, "Two Decades on, Philippines Struggles with UNITED STATES Base Cleanup," *The American Legion*, September 2012, https://hdl.handle.net/20.500.12203/4554. Accessed October, 15 2017.

10. H. G. Reza, "Navy to Stop Recruiting Filipino Nationals," *Los Angeles Times*, February 27, 1992, http://articles.latimes.com/1992-02-27/local/me-3911_1_filipino-sailors. Accessed October 20, 2017.

11. Rick Baldoz, *The Third Asiatic Invasion: Migration and Empire in Filipino America, 1898–1946* (New York: NYU Press, 2011).

12. "Filipinos in the United States Navy," Prepared by Bureau of Naval Personnel October 1976, Naval History and Heritage Command, updated September 12, 2017, https://www.history.navy.mil/research/library/online-reading-room/title-list-alphabetically/f/filipinos-in-the-united-states-navy.html.

13. Ibid.

14. Cited in Espiritu, *Home Bound: Filipino*, 30.

15. In addition to Choy, see, for example, Laura R. Prieto, "Dazzling Visions: American Women, Race and the Imperialist Origins of Modern Nursing in Cuba, 1898–1916," *Nursing History Review* 26 (2018): 116–37; Elizabeth Carnegie, "Black Nurses at the Front," *American Journal of Nursing* 84, no. 10 (October 1984): 1252; and Warwick Anderson, *Colonial Pathologies: American Tropical Medicine, Race, and Hygiene in the Philippines* (Durham: Duke University Press, 2006).

16. Choy, *Empire of Care*.

17. Ibid.

18. Maria C. Jereos, "Supply and Demand of Nurses," *Philippine Journal of Nursing* 47, no. 1 (1978): 3–5; Choy, *Empire of Care*.

19. Julite V. Sotejo, "Status of Nursing in the Philippines," *The Filipino Nurse* 20, no. 2 (January 1951): 52–55.

20. Choy, *Empire of Care*; See also Richard E. Joyce and Chester L. Hunt, "Philippine Nurses and the Brain Drain," *Social Science Medicine* 16 (1982): 1223–33.

21. Cited in Roger Daniels, *Guarding the Golden Door: American Immigration Policy and Immigrants since 1882* (New York: Hill and Wang, 2004), 165.

22. Sotejo, "Status of Nursing in the Philippines."

23. Barbara Brush, "Sending for Nurses: Foreign Nurse Immigration to American Hospitals, 1945–1980." PhD diss., University of Pennsylvania, 1994, 104, https://repository.upenn.edu/dissertations/AAI9521006. Accessed October 20, 2017.

24. "Address of His Excellency, President Ferdinand E. Marcos," *Philippine Journal of Nursing* 43 (January-March 1974): 22.

25. David Bearinger, "Filipino Traditions in Virginia," *Global Virginia, Virginia Humanities,* accessed May 30, 2018, https://www.virginiahumanities.org/2016/10/filipino-traditions-in-virginia/.

26. The Filipino American National Historical Society Hampton Roads Chapter, ed., *In Our Aunties' Words: The Filipino Spirit of Hampton Roads* (San Francisco: T'boli Publishing and Distributor, 2004).

27. Ferdinand Villamor Tolentino and John Inocian Labra, "Professions," in (Ed.,) Filipino American National Historical Society Hampton Roads Chapter. *In Our Aunties' Words: The Filipino Spirit of Hampton Roads* (San Francisco: T'boli Publishing and Distributor, 2004), 65.

28. The Filipino American National Historical Society Hampton Roads Chapter, *In Our Aunties' Words*.

29. Patricia D'Antonio, *American Nursing: A History of Knowledge, Authority, and the Meaning of Work* (Baltimore: The Johns Hopkins University Press, 2010); Hampton Roads Naval Historical Foundation, *Images of America: Naval Station Norfolk*, 101.

30. Memorandum to: Presidents and Executive Directors of State Nurses' Associations, District Nurses' Associations and State Boards of Nursing from: Doris De Vincenzo, 15 March 1968, Pennsylvania Nurses association Collection, District 1, Box 14, Folder "Immigrant Nurses, 1968," University of Pennsylvania, School of Nursing, Center for the Study of the History of Nursing Archives, quoted in Brush, "Sending for Nurses," 104.

31. Tolentino and Labra, "Professions," 67.

32. The Filipino American National Historical Society Hampton Roads Chapter, *In Our Aunties Words*.

33. Clarita Go Miraflor, "The Philippine Nurse: Implications for Orientation and in-service Education for Foreign Nurses in the United States." PhD diss., Loyola University Chicago, 1976, 58.

34. Jolly Capucao, interview by Reynaldo Capucao, Jr., October 22, 2017.

35. Norma D. Bariso, "History of the Philippine Nurses Association of Virginia, Inc.," (unpublished memorandum, September 16, 2017), private collection.

36. Lydia A. Villanueva, "Our History: The Council of United Filipino Organizations of Tidewater, Virginia Inc.," accessed May 29, 2018, http://philippineculturalcenter.com/cufot-history/.

37. Araceli Marcial, interview by Reynaldo Capucao, Jr., October 21, 2017.

Disclosure. The author has no relevant financial interest or affiliations with any commercial interests related to the subjects discussed within this article.

REYNALDO CAPUCAO JR., MSN, BA
Eleanor Crowder Bjoring
Center for Nursing Historical Inquiry
225 Jeanette Lancaster Way
University of Virginia School of Nursing
Charlottesville, Virginia

"The Force Behind the Vision": The Significance of Place in Trauma Nursing

Trina K. Kumodzi
University of Virginia

In 1960, R. Adams Cowley and Elizabeth Scanlan created the Shock Trauma Unit (STU) at the University of Maryland Medical Center in Baltimore, Maryland. As one author noted, "[Scanlan] worked side-by-side with Cowley as the first director of nursing at the STU and was considered his partner, collaborator, and friend. Cowley referred to [Scanlan] as the 'force behind the vision.'"[1] This article examines the pioneering legacy of trauma nurses from 1960 to 2000 through the conceptual lens of place. The beginning of the STU in 1960 at the University of Maryland Medical Center provides an ideal context to consider the practices, negotiations, and relationships that gave rise to a nursing specialty at a particular geographic and social place. In this case, the concept of place is not only a city or building but also a locale, or a specific setting in which people conducted their work amid a web of social relationships and assumptions about nursing and medicine within the hospital institution.[2]

Trauma nurses were a critical part of the mid-twentieth century move to establish separate spaces where they could concentrate on caring for the critically injured. They knew their nursing practice was inextricably linked to their patients' tenuous near-death status, and all would be governed by the great equalizer: time. Trauma nurses became principal healthcare professionals who worked with surgeons, physicians, and politicians to establish trauma-specific healthcare in specialized areas. Nurses were a bridge between resources and the under-resourced. Unquestionably, the success of securing state and federal funding for trauma centers depended on the work of the nurses.[3] This article moves nurses from the margins to the center of the story of trauma. Nurses, most of whom were female, and surgeons, most of whom were male, formed a distinct partnership as they developed a professional and social place that housed critically ill trauma patients.

Nursing History Review 28 (2020): 170–184. A Publication of the American Association for the History of Nursing. Copyright © 2020 Springer Publishing Company.
http://dx.doi.org/10.1891/1062-8061.28.170

To understand the context for the establishment of the STU in Baltimore, one can start in the early twentieth century. At that time, the University of Maryland created its own dispensary so that poor patients could have access to care. Over time, the University of Maryland Hospital expanded into classrooms for medical students, and they continued to use the poor as teaching subjects. After World War 1, millions of people from the rural South moved to cities further north and west, and they had a huge impact on the need for healthcare resources. Context also centers on the industrial, post-automobile city in the second half of the twentieth century. Like other large cities, Baltimore became a site for many traffic accidents and increased urban violence. Thus, more patients became available for hospital teaching in the 1960s and 1970s when the STU expanded.[4] By the 1970s, the unit provided a place for the reception of highly technical, specialized, and sophisticated care. As a teaching institution, it also was a place where patients could claim the services of experts such as Cowley and Scanlan.

Historical Background of Trauma Nursing

The STU at the University of Maryland Medical Center is one of the highest-volume trauma centers in the country. Trauma was historically situated in battlefields and in an expanding interest in civilian care after World War II.[5] War and the ensuing human suffering were incubators for much medical innovation and performance improvement. Research conducted during World War II, for example, was invaluable in identifying shock states and subsequent resuscitation of the critically wounded.[6] More extensive medical research was conducted during the Korean and Vietnam Wars, and the considerable progress in transportation, surgical procedures, and resuscitation in the field led to a reduction in death rates.[7] Whereas time to treatment was 10 hours in World War II, it dropped to half that time in the Korean War and was an incredible 1 hour in the Vietnam War.[8]

Yet wartime studies had not informed the medical treatment of civilian injuries. In 1952, to develop this line of research, President Harry S. Truman appointed George Armstrong as Surgeon General. Armstrong noted:

> Severe surgical shock following trauma is not commonly encountered in the medical practice of any group during peacetime. When it occurs it is the result of unexpected accident, and adequate provision for careful study has seldom been available. Consequently, although considerable noteworthy experimental work had been done on shock in animals since World War I, little opportunity has existed to study this serious condition in man.[9]

Traffic safety also was a major public health concern, and John F. Kennedy made it one of his platforms during his 1960 campaign for the presidency. Between 1961 and 1963 the President's Advisory Committee for Traffic Safety reported on dire traffic statistics. In 1956, for example, with 77.9 million licensed drivers and 65.2 million vehicles in the United States, 39,628 fatalities occurred. The 1960 statistics were equally bleak: fatalities totaled 38,200 with one and a half million injuries and billions of dollars in lost property attributable to lack of traffic safety.[10] The staggering human and financial cost of injury was slowly infiltrating the American consciousness.[11]

Survivors of accidents and violence became ever present in large city hospitals, and these evolved into places for a new kind of healthcare professional, the trauma nurse. Much of the literature in this field focuses on male doctors and surgeons, especially since the trauma specialty is renowned for its fast pace and complex technological interventions.[12] As Julie Fairman and Joan Lynaugh assert, however, nurses have played a crucial role in shaping and delivering care in critical care sites that are integral to America's complex healthcare delivery system today.[13] Perhaps the most paradoxical aspect of the nurse–physician relationship in such highly technical places as trauma units is the dissolution of the gendered interactions prevalent in nurse–physician communication throughout the rest of the hospital. In the STU, social and professional interactions mediated specific power structures. Examining the work of nurses validates their contribution to the trauma specialty in places where nurses and physicians worked together in their efforts to heal patients.

The STU as a Case Study for Place in Trauma Nursing

Baltimore's explosive growth after World War II led enterprising physicians and nurses to establish new sites for critical care. The University of Maryland Medical Center became a mecca for meeting the needs of survivors of violence and traffic accidents. In 1960, the Army awarded a $100,000 grant to fund Cowley to do research on shock. Cowley was a cardiothoracic surgeon in the hospital, having practiced and done research in post–World War II Europe. This two-bed research unit, the STU, was nicknamed the Death Lab because of the unit's initially high death rate. Soon it expanded to four beds and became the first civilian trauma center in the United States.[14] As clinical outcomes improved, confidence in the unit grew, largely due to the expert nursing care that developed at that time, led by Scanlan.

In 1957, Scanlan graduated from the St. Agnes Hospital School of Nursing in Baltimore and started working as a nurse at the University of Maryland Medical Center. By 1960, she had earned her master's degree from the University of Maryland School of Nursing.[15] Scanlan and Cowley quickly became collaborators. As a wartime surgeon, Cowley had observed patients in shock, and he developed a theoretical method to save them: both speed and skill were the two crucial elements. He coined the term, the "Golden Hour," that hour "between life and death. If you are critically injured you have less than 60 minutes to survive. You might not die right then; it may be three days or two weeks later—but something has happened in your body that is irreparable."[16]

This was particularly the case with gunshot wounds, and clinicians increasingly recognized the need for faster streamlined care. In 1963, a physician and two nurses wrote an *American Journal of Nursing* article that cited National Safety Council's firearm-related civilian injury statistics from 1900 to 1960. They showed little to no change in the medical care of the survivors. To these authors, this "would certainly suggest that more attention needs to be paid to the factors leading to gunshot injuries."[17] While skills were important, time and place of treatment were critical factors.

The STU was significant not only for patients who received expert care but also for the personnel who worked in the unit. As Fairman and Lynaugh note, the nurses in the new intensive care units of the 1960s were often the most experienced and knowledgeable in the hospital. Scanlan was one of those nurses. The STU became an ideal setting for new nurse–physician alliances that expanded the boundaries of authority for nurses. As they worked quickly and skillfully in the units, nurses gained what Fairman and Lynaugh call a "zone of authority," which gave them the opportunity to use their unique expertise.[18] Furthermore, as patients grew in complexity, their conditions demanded a "new way of thinking." At the same time, skilled nurses were growing in number as graduate nurses at the bedside replaced student labor.[19] These highly skilled and knowledgeable nurses, concentrated in small areas of intensive care units such as the STU, provided a much more stable environment for patients, which also reassured physicians and increased their respect for nurses.[20] These were the contextual forces in which collaboration and respect became the foundation of the nurse–doctor relationship for Scanlan and Cowley in the STU. Their relationship was the prototype that the other nurses and physicians emulated throughout the hospital.

The development of a robust national trauma center in Baltimore was contingent upon federal funding and legislation.[21] In 1966, the National Academy of Sciences National Research Council created a task force, the Committee on Trauma and the Committee on Shock. It wrote the white paper, *Accidental*

Death and Disability: The Neglected Disease of Modern Society, the first major federal document recognizing civilian-based injury and trauma, its human and financial costs, and the lack of infrastructure and trained personnel to effectively prevent and treat it.[22] Injury, trauma, and the subsequent disability discussions had percolated in silos throughout the country, and the *Accidental Death and Disability* report galvanized the individuals into a collective that signaled it was time to do something. President Lyndon B. Johnson signed the Highway Safety Act into law on September 9, 1966, saying: "Safety is no luxury item, it is no optional extra; it must be a normal cost of doing business."[23] The Act allocated federal funds toward highway safety: $50 million for fiscal year 1966, $80 million for fiscal year 1967, $85 million for fiscal year 1968, $110 million for fiscal year 1969, $115 million for fiscal year 1970, and $140 million for fiscal year 1971.[24] The National Highway Safety Bureau (which became the National Highway Traffic Safety Administration in 1970) subsequently took over fund management and disbursement. The Highway Safety Act of 1966 allocated specific funds for improved medical services in specialized places with highly trained personnel.[25]

Financing from other federal agencies soon became available. The Alcohol, Drug Abuse, and Mental Health Administration (ADAMHA), Health Services Administration (HSA), Comprehensive Health Planning Service (CHPS), Health Resources Administration (HRA), and the Regional Medical Program Service (RMPS) funded emergency medical service (EMS) projects. The Emergency Medical Services Act of 1973 was the pioneering legislation that established federal funding strictly for improved and more accessible EMS. One hundred and ninety million dollars went to state-run EMS over 3 years.[26] All of these grants were contingent upon a qualified emergency medical system that included special care units. The goal was to reduce the nation's disability and death statistics through federal mandates of a systems approach at the regional level for emergency care response.[27] The Act underwent revision in 1976 as the Emergency Medical Services Amendments (Public Law 94–573) to fund statewide EMS services in medically underserved regions across the nation.[28] As well, Medicare and Medicaid had become law in 1965, and these programs became crucial sources of government payments to both public and private facilities. Settings such as the STU could pass expenses not only to the government but also to insurance companies such as Blue Cross and Blue Shield, which had been expanding since the 1930s. This expansive time certainly benefited the STU.

Nursing in the STU

New treatments, new facilities, and new money meant a new era for nurses as clinical partners. As federal funding became more available, trauma systems as specialized places were not static. Scanlan wrote grant proposals for the unit and secured a National Institutes of Health grant for expansion.[29] In 1969 the 5-story, 32-bed Center for the Study of Trauma opened. Cowley and Scanlan also formulated a plan for a statewide helicopter evacuation program. The Maryland Air Medevac Helicopter System, the nation's first such program, developed in 1969 in a joint partnership with the University of Maryland Center for the Study of Trauma.[30]

The emergency department, trauma unit, and other medical systems became places for innovative and expansive nursing roles. Arlene Keeling asserts, "In the 1960s, the invisible boundary separating the permissible from the non-permissible in the practice of medicine and nursing was blurring."[31] The trauma nursing specialty considerably improved the care of complex and critically injured patients to heights unwitnessed in most medical centers. Bedside trauma nurses, nurse specialists, and coordinator roles were integral in advancing consistent, reliable, and superior-quality hospital care within regional trauma systems such as the STU.[32] Mary Beachley, an influential trauma nurse pioneer, explained nursing's position in both the trauma hospital and the patient's recovery: "Nursing is the cornerstone of the hospital's trauma program. Nursing's challenge is to provide a continuum of nursing care that meets the urgent, complex needs of the trauma patient and family from time of injury through rehabilitation and reintegration into the community."[33]

As complex care became more medically specialized, nursing care was the only constant in the patient's treatment. Services in orthopedic surgery, plastic surgery, critical care, infectious disease, neurosurgery, oral surgery, interventional radiology, and traumatology grew. Medical care fragmented according to expertise and became isolated from the problems and injuries affecting the person. Because trauma patients had many injuries to different body regions, each injury necessitated interventions geared toward survival and recovery.[34] For example, a patient suffering from a motor vehicle collision might have orthopedic, neurological, and cardiac surgeries in addition to separate medical consults from renal, infectious disease, hepatic, and pulmonology physicians. All congregated in trauma units, and nurses became the key facilitators and coordinators in this multidisciplinary care network.

The meaning of place and identity for nursing was indeed changing in the 1960s. Keeling chronicled the expansion of nursing's role at this time:

Since each minute of delay could be life-threatening, autonomy in decision making during those emergencies was essential. So was the authority to treat the patient . . . What was new was the fact that nurses had to move from simply collecting data and reporting their findings, as they had long been doing when they took temperatures and blood pressures, to acting on their own assessment of the data when necessary, prior to reporting it to a physician. In essence, the nurses expanded their roles to include curing as well as caring.[35]

Betty Jane Tarrant was another nurse instrumental in the development of the trauma nurse specialty. As the nurse supervisor in the University of Maryland Center for the Study of Trauma, she promoted the innovative work of the Center through her conference presentations and journal articles. At the November 1965 American Nurses Association (ANA) Conference, for example, she presented the therapeutic treatments for shock to the attending nurses. She highlighted the critical decision-making skills of the nurse in trauma units when she explained that "the nurse regulates the infusion rate by watching the central venous pressure and its relation to the blood pressure." Tarrant asserted to her ANA colleagues that more shock-trauma centers would soon open across the country, particularly in the university hospital setting.[36] Tarrant's clinical research centered on what she referred to as "automation," the patient's experience within the technological intrusions of trauma care. In her 1966 *American Journal of Nursing* article, "Automation: Its Effect on the Patient," she outlined a specific role for how nurses could be the best ones to help:

Automation is an 'explosive force'- an important and far-reaching extension of technological advances already effected in this century. It has become an integral part of the hospital environment. But how does it affect the hospitalized patient and the nurse who cares for him? . . . The use of automation in hospitals continues to grow. Its influence upon patient therapy, patients as people, nursing, and nurses will need to be continually evaluated . . . Studies must be made that will enable us to identify how best to help a patient accept and integrate into his life an experience of dependency on a machine. We have to remember machines are useful only to the extent of our knowledge and ability to utilize them for the welfare of our patients: that human observation and judgment must always precede their use, and then continue to determine their value to the patient.[37]

Tarrant's concerns reflect the trauma nurse's zeal for cutting-edge therapy tempered with a holistic respect for the patient. It was in the electronic clinical environment of the STU that her work could advance both the technology and the human experience as a nurse.

In this atmosphere, Scanlan and Tarrant became what many consider the nation's first trauma-specialty nurses, working tirelessly at the bedside, writing grants, teaching students, and publishing articles in peer-reviewed journals. As master's-prepared nurses, they used their clinical skills and keen intelligence to expand the boundaries of nursing.[38] Scanlan instituted trauma nurse specialty tenets and regionalized trauma and critical nurse education programs.

Although federal funding to emergency services decreased during the Reagan Administration, other funds had become available for graduate programs in nursing. Thus, Scanlan was able to establish the University of Maryland School of Nursing's Critical Care and Trauma Nursing master's program in 1985. She mentored many influential and renowned trauma nurse coordinators, including Virginia Cardona, Peggy Trimble, and Carol Katsaras. The STU expanded again 1989 and was renamed the R. Adams Cowley Shock Trauma Center (STC), a freestanding eight-story, 113-bed state-of-the-art facility. As the Director of Nursing, Scanlan was instrumental in the architectural design for the facility.[39]

The Power of Place in Nursing History

In thinking about the power of place in nursing history, nowhere was this more evident than in the STU in Baltimore. Nurses relished their prominence in this trauma specialty. In their "zone of authority," nurses had a level of autonomy they had not experienced in other areas of the hospital.[40] They proudly wore the shocking pink-colored scrubs that identified them as members of the STU team. The uniforms not only set up hierarchies among nurses, but they also set nurses apart as skilled workers in a very special place. Protocols, the established clinical guidelines for the treatment management of a particular condition, gave the nurses latitude to practice to their training's fullest extent. As B.J. Breeze, a nurse in STU, commented:

> We know the protocols very well down here . . . We know the hierarchy of priorities, the Advanced Trauma Life Support, and our own admitting area protocols. With all that, we don't miss much. Everybody has a designated task or set of tasks . . . I don't have to stand there and tell the resident, "Now you do this"; anesthesia doesn't have to tell me, "Get a blood pressure and the ABGs."[41]

Trauma nurses thrived in this place of collegial and intellectual stimulation.

Nursing administration equally prospered in this type of clinical setting. Colleen Walleck, the STU's Associate Director of Nursing, described innovative nursing research ideas and projects:

One of the early projects grew out of complaints by neuro nurses about products they used for Foley care. [We] helped them design a protocol that compared the effectiveness of plain soap and water for Foley care against some fancy product that cost a fortune. All the neuro nurses had to do was document their regular nursing care. If they used a Foley kit, they wrote "K" in a space after "Foley care," and if not, they left the space blank. A staff nurse collected the data at the end of each shift, and we compared it to results from the routine urine cultures done twice a week. We found no significant difference between soap and water and the kit. And the staff got a $50 reward for the cost-containment effort.[42]

Clearly, survival of growing numbers of critically injured people depended on access to the highly skilled and technical care available in a trauma unit.

On February 26, 1973, Maryland Governor Marvin Mandel issued an executive order that renamed the University of Maryland Center for the Study of Trauma as the Maryland Institute for Emergency Medicine. The Maryland Institute for Emergency Medicine Services Systems (MIEMSS) became the first statewide EMS system in the nation.[43] Nurses were key contributors to the development of the prehospital care-to-hospital model. For example, they educated EMS providers in effective prehospital care. Annie Smith Rehfeld's collaboration with Cowley to set training standards for EMS flight personnel is an example. She led resuscitation nurses in the hands-on skills and didactic training for the Aviation Trauma Technician (ATT) program.[44] In 1975, Scanlan established the MIEMSS Field Nursing program. This program provided seminars and workshops covering more than 50 EMS and trauma topics for nurses in Maryland. In 1982, Trimble, Scanlan's mentee, developed and became the Director for the MIEMSS Field Nursing Program. Within this program, she and her staff created the Advanced Trauma Life Support for Nurses continuing education course.[45] Trimble also collaborated with Lou Jordan, a former military corpsman, to create a similar education program for statewide training for Maryland's EMS providers.[46]

Scanlan retired in 1989.[47] Her importance is evident in an article written by a nurse that year in the *American Journal of Nursing*:

If Cowley's vision of the "golden hour" became the prototype for peacetime shock trauma care, his dependence on and respect for Elizabeth Scanlan, Shock Trauma's first nurse and now its director of nursing, was the prototype for the mutual respect and collaboration between nurses and physicians at MIEMSS. According to Scanlan, Dr. Cowley was quick to appreciate the importance of the nurse's ability to make acute observations, to notice subtle changes, to assess trends, and to act quickly on those judgments. More than that, he relied on her vision as much as his own.[48]

As this nurse described it, the STU was a place of social interactions and collaborations created by both nurses and physicians. Scanlan stated: "We created this environment together. Our concept was to handle trauma from the scene of injury all the way to rehabilitation. We wrote the grants together, went to government officials for funding, and fought with hospital boards to get the staff we needed. The atmosphere here today grew from that."[49] Her words say a great deal about units such as the STU, where new socialization patterns developed. Thus, supporting Fairman and Lynaugh' assertions, the STU served as "a testing ground on which a more collaborative structure was explored and found to be beneficial."[50]

Trauma Nurses and Professionalization

As nurses helped create this special place, they also used it as a site for greater professionalization of trauma nursing. Nurses' influence and power were growing within all aspects of trauma care, and they recognized the need for a more efficient means of sharing information within the profession. Nurses attending the 1983 MIEMSS National Trauma Symposium recognized the need for a formal network. Thus, they led the establishment of the Trauma Nurse Network (TNN) in 1986 with financial support from MIEMSS. Biannual meetings convened during the National Trauma Symposium and the California Trauma Conference. In June 1988, the TNN published its newsletter complete with a consensus statement detailing the definition of trauma nursing, its philosophy, and standards. The September 1988 edition included the consensus statement on trauma nursing education and designation. The publication reached an impressive 1,500 members.[51] The Emergency Department Nurses Association (currently the Emergency Nurses Association), founded in 1970, offered the first Trauma Nursing Core Course, the entry-level course for trauma nurse credentialing at that time.[52]

In 1989, as its recognition expanded, the TNN organized a national professional organization, the Society of Trauma Nurses (STN). In 1990, members elected Mary Beachley, who had served as the Maryland state representative in the TNN, as the organization's first president.[53] Thereafter, the STN gained prominence as the premier trauma nursing organization and possessed both the intellect and clout to change policy. For example, it collaborated with many national and governmental organizations such as the Health Resources and Services Administration's 1992 *Model Trauma System Care Plan*. Nurses in the STN also helped write the Trauma Coordinator section of the

American College of Surgeons Committee on Trauma's *Resources for Optimal Care of the Injured Patient.*[54] The 1994 inaugural issue of *Journal of Trauma Nursing* became the platform to disseminate evidence-based knowledge to trauma practitioners. Originally the STN held its meetings during the National Trauma Care Symposium and the Trauma Society's Modern Concepts in Trauma Symposium. By 1998, however, the STN had the structural and organizational infrastructure in place to hold its inaugural Annual STN Conference in Las Vegas, Nevada. By 1999, STN membership totaled 303 members.[55]

In 2011, David R. Boyd, founder of the trauma unit at the Cook County Hospital in Chicago and one of Cowley's first medical residents in the University of Maryland Center for the Study of Trauma, noted: "A national consensus now asserts: the 'Trauma EMS Systems Approach' to improved trauma care works! There are volumes of confirmatory publications on positive outcomes and evidence of the effectiveness of trauma centers and trauma systems." He then noted something else that speaks to the sense of locale and belonging so fundamental to nurses who work in intensive care units: "The trauma nurses . . . are absolutely essential 'players' in this great story . . ."[56]

A growing urban population paralleled the growth of hospitals in the early twentieth century, and this movement continued into the 1960s and 1970s as the federal government increasingly focused on civilian-based injuries and trauma units. In this context, both nurses and physicians collaborated to establish important places for care. In the trauma unit, place involved not only a specific area where patients could get expert care but also a site for the development of a special meaning for the nurses who worked in the units: an increasing feeling of attachment, value, collaboration, and authority. Nurses strongly believed that patient care depended on experts in specialized units such as the STU, and contemporary units continue to give visibility to nurses' distinct roles. In rehabilitating the prominence of place in nursing history, it is important to add that national recognition of the necessity coupled with technologic growth and nurse advocacy created these specialized places.[57] As Rashidah B. Fransisco, a nurse on the MIEMSS' Lung Rescue Unit explains:

> When asking myself where I could go to be a part of the best, where only the best is expected of me, and where my skills and education would be the only determining factor in how far I can go in my career, I chose Shock Trauma [STC]. I have been at STC for over 4 years, and there is not one day that I have not been pleased with my career choice . . . Wearing the pink uniform is something that for the last four years I have been very proud of. It is to me like putting an "S" on my chest when getting ready for my shift. However, it is something that comes with a heavy responsibility and a possession of skills that I am expected to have and use when I walk through the

doors of STC. My days are not blissful, my days are not easy, but they have been more rewarding at STC than they have my entire nursing career.[58]

Her words validate an understanding of what place as both a physical location and locale mean, and they speak to what Charles W. J. Withers describes: "place [is] a consequence not just of emotional attachments in and to a setting," but also of "the importance of the lived experiences and embodied practices there."[59] To Fransisco, it was in the STU that these experiences developed, not elsewhere.

Notes

1. Dan Caughey, "Pioneers in Trauma: How a Doctor/Nurse Team Established Trauma Care as a Medical Specialty," *The Magazine of the University of Maryland School of Nursing* 6, no. 2 (2012): 16–17. Quotation is on page 17.

2. John A. Agnew, James S. Duncan, eds., *The Power of Place: Bringing Together Geographical and Sociological Imaginations* (London: Routledge, 1989, 2013).

3. Priscilla Scherer, "Shock Trauma," *The American Journal of Nursing* 89, no. 11 (1989): 1440–45, accessed October 5, 2015, http://www.jstor.org/stable/3426144. Accessed October 5, 2015

4. Charles E. Rosenberg, *The Care of Strangers: The Rise of America's Hospital System* (Baltimore: Johns Hopkins University Press, 1995).

5. Karen McQuillan et al., *Trauma Nursing: From Resuscitation through Rehabilitation*, 3rd ed. (Philadelphia: W.B. Saunders, 2002), 4; Jody Foss, "A History of Trauma Care: From Cutter to Surgeon," *AORN Journal* 50, no. 1 (1989): 28; Richard J. Mullins, "A Historical Perspective of Trauma System Development in the United States," *Journal of Trauma: Injury, Infection, and Critical Care* 47, no. 3 (1999): S9–S12.

6. Board for the Study of the Severely Wounded North African-Mediterranean Theater of Operations, Medical Department, United States Army. *Surgery in World War II: The Physiologic effect of Wounds* (Washington, DC: U.S. Government Printing Office, 1952), 1–5, accessed October 19, 2015, https://collections.nlm.nih.gov/ext/dw/101142056/PDF/101142056.pdf

7. McQuillan et al., *Trauma Nursing*, 4.

8. David Boyd and R. Adams Cowley, "Comprehensive Regional Trauma/Emergency Medical Services (EMS) Delivery Systems: The United States Experience," *World Journal of Surgery* 7, no. 1 (1983): 151.

9. Cited in Board for the Study of the Severely Wounded, *Surgery in World War II*, 5.

10. Papers of John F. Kennedy. Presidential Papers. President's Office Files. Departments and Agencies. Committee for Traffic Safety, 15 January 1962–23 October 1963. doi:JFKPOF-093-011.

11. McQuillan et al., *Trauma Nursing*, 3–5.

12. An Amazon.com search for "nursing history books" yielded 35,000 titles. The first 80 titles were screened for duplicates and irrelevant books. This resulted in 15 relevant nursing history titles.

13. Julie Fairman and Joan Lynaugh, *Critical Care Nursing: A History* (Philadelphia: University of Pennsylvania Press, 1998), 15–20, 112–18.

14. "History of the Shock Trauma Center: Tribute to R. Adams Cowley, M.D.," University of Maryland Medical Center, accessed November 1, 2015, http://umm.edu/programs/shock-trauma/about/history.

15. Frederick N. Rasmussen, "The Obituary of Elizabeth S. Trump," *The Baltimore Sun*, June 9, 2012, accessed November 7, 2015, http://www.baltimoresun.com/news/obituaries/bs-md-ob-elizabeth-trump-20120608-story.html.

16. "History of the Shock Trauma Center." See also Scherer, "Shock Trauma."

17. Leonard Worman, Carol Yount, and Lois Jacobs, "The Care of Patients with Gunshot Wounds," *The American Journal of Nursing* 63, no. 2 (1963): 93–96, accessed October 30, 2015, http://www.jstor.org/stable/3452604. Quotation is on page 93. Accessed October 30, 2015

18. Fairman and Lynaugh, *Critical Care Nursing*, 78.

19. Ibid., 77.

20. Ibid., 87–88.

21. Mary Beachley and Sandra Snow, "Developing Trauma Care Systems: A Nursing Perspective," *The Journal of Nursing Administration* 18, no. 4 (1988): 22–23.

22. Committee on Trauma and Committee on Shock, *Accidental Death and Disability: The Neglected Disease of Modern Society* (Washington, DC: National Academy of Sciences, 1966), 5–6, accessed October 25, 2015, http://www.nap.edu/read/9978/chapter/1.

23. Lyndon B. Johnson, "Remarks at the Signing of the National Traffic and Motor Vehicle Safety Act and the Highway Safety Act," September 9, 1966; Online by Gerhard Peters and John T. Woolley, "The American Presidency Project," accessed October 25, 2015, http://www.presidency.ucsb.edu/node/238669

24. Committee on Public Works, *Highway Safety Act of 1966: Hearings before the United States House Committee on Public Works, Eighty-Ninth Congress, Second Session, on Mar. 22–24, May 3–5, 1966* (Washington, DC, 1966), 3, accessed December 14, 2018, https://catalog.hathitrust.org/Record/008467049.

25. Ibid., 7.

26. Committee on Interstate and Foreign Commerce, *Emergency Medical Services Act of 1973: Hearing before the Subcommittee on Public Health and Environment of the Committee on Interstate and Foreign Commerce House of Representatives, Ninety-Third Congress, First Session* (Washington, DC: Government Printing Office, 1973), 1.

27. McQuillan et al., *Trauma Nursing*, 6.

28. Mullins, "A Historical Perspective."

29. Caughey, "Pioneers in Trauma"; Rasmussen, "The Obituary of Elizabeth S. Trump"; Scherer, "Shock Trauma," 1442.

30. R. Adams Cowley et al., "An Economical and Proved Helicopter Program for Transporting the Emergency Critically Ill and Injured Patient in Maryland," *Journal of Trauma* 13, no. 12 (1973): 1029.

31. Arlene W. Keeling, "Blurring the Boundaries Between Medicine and Nursing: Coronary Care Nursing, Circa the 1960s," *Nursing History Review* 12 (2004): 139–64. Quotation is on page 139.

32. David R. Boyd, "Trauma Nurses: Historical Notes and Appreciation," *Journal of Trauma Nursing* 18, no. 3 (2011): 187; Beachley and Snow, "Developing Trauma Care Systems."

33. Beachley and Snow, "Developing Trauma Care Systems," 26.

34. Mullins, "A Historical Perspective."

35. Keeling, "Blurring the Boundaries," 156.

36. "Clinical Conference Focus: The Nurse is One Who Cares," *American Journal of Nursing* 66, no. 1 (1966): 12.

37. Betty Jane Tarrant, "Automation: Its Effect on the Patient," *The American Journal of Nursing* 66, no. 10 (1966): 2190–94, accessed October 12, 2015, http://www.jstor.org/stable/3419986. Quotation is on pages 2190 and 2194. Accessed October 12, 2015

38. "The University of Maryland School of Nursing Catalog, 1966–1967," accessed December 4, 2018, https://www.nursing.umaryland.edu/media/son/academics/registration–records/verifications/School-of-Nursing-Catalog-1966-1970-web.pdf.

39. Caughey, "Pioneers in Trauma," 17.

40. Fairman and Lynaugh, *Critical Care Nursing*, 78.

41. Quoted in Scherer, "Shock Trauma," 1442.

42. Ibid., 1444.

43. Cowley et al., "An Economical and Proved Helicopter Program," 1029.

44. Lewis M. Flint, *Trauma: Contemporary Principles and Therapy* (Philadelphia: Wolters Kluwer Health/Lippincott Williams & Wilkins, 2008).

45. Mary Beachley, "The Evolution of Trauma Nursing and the Society of Trauma Nurses: A Noble History," *Journal of Trauma Nursing* 12, no. 4 (2005): 112.

46. Flint, *Trauma: Contemporary Principles and Therapy*, 229.

47. Scanlan was posthumously awarded one of the inaugural University of Maryland School of Nursing Visionary Pioneer Award at the University's 125th anniversary gala in April 2015. See "University of Maryland School of Nursing Announces Inaugural Visionary Pioneer Award Winners," October 16, 2014, accessed December 15, 2018, https://www.nursing.umaryland.edu/news-events/news/visionary.php. See also Boyd, "Trauma Nurses"; and Rasmussen, "The Obituary of Elizabeth S. Trump."

48. Scherer, "Shock Trauma," 1442.

49. Ibid.

50. Fairman and Lynaugh, *Critical Care Nursing*, 78.

51. Beachley, "The Evolution of Trauma Nursing."

52. Flint, *Trauma: Contemporary Principles and Therapy*.

53. Beachley, "The Evolution of Trauma Nursing."

54. Society of Trauma Nurses, "Society of Trauma Nurses Strategic Plan, 2010–2012," accessed November 2, 2015, http://www.traumanurses.org/_resources/documents/about/STN%20Strategic%20Plan%202010-2012%20Final.pdf.

55. Ibid.

56. Boyd, "Trauma Nurses: Historical Notes and Appreciation."

57. McQuillan et al., *Trauma Nursing*, 16.

58. Quoted by Michele Wojciechowski, "View from a Nurse in Shock Trauma," *Minority Nurse*, August 1, 2017, accessed May 14, 2018, https://minoritynurse.com/view-from-a-nurse-in-shock-trauma/.

59. Charles W. J. Withers, "Place and the 'Spatial' Turn in Geography and in History," *Journal of the History of Ideas* 70, no. 4 (October 2009): 637–58. Quotation is on page 658.

Disclosure. The author has no relevant financial interest or affiliations with any commercial interests related to the subjects discussed within this article.

TRINA K. KUMODZI, BSN, RN, CCRN
University of Virginia
School of Nursing
McLeod Hall
202 Jeanette Lancaster Way
Charlottesville, VA 22908

NOTES AND DOCUMENTS

"The Ambulances Are Running in Every Direction": A Patient's Experience of Influenza in a Military Camp, 1918

Janet Golden
Rutgers University–Camden

Twenty-one-year-old Corporal Alton W. Miller died of pneumonia following influenza in the base hospital at Camp Zachary Taylor, in Louisville, Kentucky, on October 11, 1918. He was one of more than a million Army men to contract influenza prior to going overseas and one of 43,000 men in uniform to die.[1] What makes his death remarkable is its documentation. His family kept a scrapbook with typed transcriptions of his letters recounting his illness and, after his death, a letter reporting on his last hours. An unidentified nurse, present at the death of Miller, portrayed the efforts made to save his life and conveyed the details of his death to his close friend.[2]

The collection of letters from Miller and from other men in uniform provides a compelling portrait of the lived experience of influenza at a time when there were no effective means of prevention and limited treatments for this massive and seemingly unstoppable disease outbreak. They not only detail the care given to patients and the demise of Corporal Miller and others, they also serve to remind us of how influenza mortality in the early twentieth century was explained in medical terms while comfort to the bereaved often came through religious expressions. The germ theory transformed medical practice in the early twentieth century but it did not change the way death was understood.

Nursing History Review 28 (2020): 185–195. A Publication of the American Association for the History of Nursing. Copyright © 2020 Springer Publishing Company.
http://dx.doi.org/10.1891/1062-8061.28.185

Large-scale studies of the 1918–1919 pandemic reveal the enormity of sickness and loss, with an estimated 50 million deaths worldwide and 650,000 in the United States. There are scholarly accounts of the epidemic within nations and communities, of the flu's effects on the course of World War I, of its impact on public health systems, and of efforts to halt the spread of the epidemic.[3] Newspaper records, oral histories from survivors, and literary accounts provide additional insights. Eyewitness accounts, such as the one presented by Corporal Miller and his friend, offer a different vantage point, revealing how influenza narratives could resemble earlier depictions of illness and death in their religious rhetoric while also showing how patients experienced disease. The accounts reveal what ordinary people thought about in the midst of the epidemic, how they attempted to avoid becoming ill, and how they responded when influenza struck.[4] Corporal Miller's letters as well as others from members of the military make clear that despite the relatively recent experience of the 1889–1890 pandemic that took 1 million lives, the US military, the nation, and the world was unprepared for the 1918 outbreak. And they soon learned that it was deadliest among young adults.

Scholars view the epidemic as sparking a transition in the practice of medicine and public health. Disease containment, improved sanitation, vaccine trials and assessment, disaster planning, community education, and new knowledge about disease all followed in the wake of the influenza pandemic.[5] But what should not be lost to scholars were the ways eighteenth and nineteenth century American experiences with disease and death shaped religious expressions of comfort to the grief-stricken families.

Corporal Miller

Twenty-one year old Alton Miller worked as a chauffeur in his hometown of Kingston, New York, until July 24, 1918 when he reported to the New York State Armory in Kingston and then, 2 days later to Camp Dix, New Jersey where he began his training, along with many other draftees from his hometown. During World War I men from the same community often served together. As a result, the letters sent home by soldiers and sailors often reported on friends and acquaintances known to their families. Shortly after his departure, Miller wrote to his sister that about 100 "fellows from Kingston" were sent home as physically unfit but about 140 others remained in the camp. One close hometown friend, Walton Fitzgerald, would report on Miller's final hours.[6]

Corporal Miller spent a month in training at Camp Dix. Then, newly promoted to the rank of Corporal, he wrote home to say that he would be entering Officers Training School for Artillery. His training began a few weeks later when he arrived at the newly built Camp Taylor. As medical historians observed, the frequent reposting of men and their transfer on crowded troop trains helped to spread the infection from camp to camp. Influenza arrived at Camp Dix on September 18. The outbreak at Camp Taylor began on September 22, shortly after Miller' arrival. Approximately 11,000 men posted to Camp Taylor would fall ill and an estimated 1,500 would perish.[7]

An early letter from Miller mentioned a quarantine at Camp Taylor although, he reported, it was not very strict. His letters home did not make clear who was in charge of health at the Camp and how the authorities there made decisions during the outbreak. Some military camps imposed a quarantine to keep the men from carrying the disease into nearby communities; others did not let the men leave for fear that they would acquire the disease while outside the camp. For example, as the epidemic ebbed at the Naval Hospital in Pelham Bay Park, New York, one man wrote to his father that only the hospital men were getting liberty "because of the condition outside" while others remained on base. Since he worked in the hospital he explained that he could leave camp but anyone who did so was forbidden from using the subway.[8] Social distancing through the closing of amusement centers and schools, the banning of public gatherings, and the wearing of masks were among the most common efforts undertaken in civilian areas in a failed attempt to halt the epidemic. In Miller's case, he and others were forbidden to leave camp but were free to wander about the grounds. However, he further elaborated in a letter that he could not have gone even if permitted because "We have been here eleven days and have not received our uniforms yet."[9] The lack of preparation, supplies, and organization in the hastily organized military camps would prove to be deadly when the epidemic arrived.

Letters home from other military men described the transformation of military buildings into wards as the toll of illness climbed and also revealed their fears of death.[10] "This influenza is no joke" one sailor aboard a ship docked in Newport, Rhode Island explained in a letter. The camps and stations "are full of it," he wrote, and "they are carrying a few men off the ships and they don't live over four days."[11] Conditions were no better overseas. Writing from Brest, France, a soldier told his twin sister he was sorry to learn of a death at home "but if you could of seen them drop off like I did over here you would have been so use (sic) to it that you would never looked around when they would kick the bucket, as high as twenty a night . . ."[12] Writing to his Aunt from Fort Bliss, Texas, a man explained that there were "about twenty military funerals a day" later observing of his hometown friends "about ten of our fellows have had the Spanish influenza but all have got well."[13] Documenting his recovery in the hospital at Camp McClellan in Alabama, a private observed the waning number of cases on his integrated ward "In our room we only have five of us now. Three whites and two negroes."[14]

After the United States entered the war in April 1917, the military hastily erected training camps for the men. Most of the camps lacked adequate hospital facilities able to care for the thousands who would be stricken with influenza. Physicians and nurses sent overseas for the war effort led to a shortage of stateside healthcare providers and contributed to the problem of delivering medical treatment to soldiers and sailors sickened with influenza. Patients receiving care at Camp Taylor would rely on nurses requisitioned by military leaders, Red Cross volunteers, and nurse volunteers from seven Catholic congregations, only 10 of 88 of them who were trained nurses. Aides and community volunteers also helped out in the camp hospital.[15]

Letters Home

Military leaders in the United States and overseas fighting the war made efforts to halt the spread of what was an obvious contagious respiratory ailment. Health experts endorsed masks as well as nasal and throat sprays as effective preventatives and the military made use of them. A man stationed in France reported he felt shaky but kept spraying his throat, perhaps convinced to take every precaution because, he explained, 25% of the regiment was sick.[16] Another soldier told of having to gargle before meals with a medicine that "tastes like quicklime and is very bitter" but he believed that it would keep him from getting sick. His faith seems misplaced because the evidence that it didn't work was right in front of him. Others from his hometown, Ironton, Ohio, had come down with the flu and several were in the hospital, he reported in his letter.[17] Those spared from disease credited camp prevention efforts. After describing the regimen used at his military Balloon School in Arcadia, California a soldier suggested to his family members that they adopt his regimen and use a nasal and throat spray a couple of times a day. He believed it worked because, he explained to them, Camp Dick, an aviation training facility in Texas had hundreds of cases and was under quarantine and both nearby Los Angeles and Pasadena were "full of it," but there were no cases in Arcadia where the sprays were in use.[18]

In an October 5 letter to his father Miller described his bout with the flu then making its way through the camp, but assured him he would be fine.

"Don't get frightened but I have had the Influenza for four days but I have not let the authorities know about it yet. I think I can bring myself around if I can keep up long enough." At that point, Miller had little to say about his symptoms except that "it takes the life right out of you. For a couple of days I thought I would keel over every other step." He concluded his letter "Am going to lie down for while." Evidently the outbreak was severe by that point; the authorities cancelled all passes and furloughs to prevent spreading the disease to the surrounding community.[19]

Despite his symptoms, Miller did not report his illness to his superiors because he feared entering the hospital, which he described as overcrowded. The camp hospital offered "'rotten' treatment," he wrote, having learned "It is so overcrowded that you don't get enough to eat and it is very dirty and most of the nurses and attendants have got it too." It is unclear whether Miller feared hospitals in general, as many people did in the early twentieth century because of their lingering reputation as houses of death, or whether his reluctance to seek inpatient care reflected particular conditions at the camp hospital.[20]

Another point in the letter is worth nothing. While Miller observed the dire conditions at Camp Taylor, he did not understand the extent to which the outbreak gripped the nation. 195,000 Americans would die of the flu in October 1918 and hundreds of thousands more fell ill.[21] Yet, he asked in his letter home, "Are there any cases in Kingston?" It is possible that his family kept that information from him when they wrote. The flu did reach Kingston and the local newspaper tracked the epidemic, reported on deaths, and printed articles providing (useless) health advice. Evidently concern was so high that an advertisement for workers for a sewing factory in town promised conditions were sanitary with "Airiness, sunlight, cleanliness. All tending to protect girls' health against the flu."[22]

Miller's inquiry was not surprising. In some letters exchanged between men in the military and their families they reported to each other on the explosion of cases in the camps, surrounding communities, and hometowns. In other letters, however, the men asked their families if they had heard of the flu or if it had struck back home. In their exchanges families and military men provided the names of those who had died, but with limited descriptions of their illnesses and deaths. Knowledge of the horrific and rapid deaths of hundreds of thousands of soldiers in World War I battles may have blunted the response to the more numerous, somewhat slower though relentless toll of stateside and overseas deaths from pneumonia following influenza.

The personnel at Camp Taylor, like those in other military facilities and across the nation, sickened and died at an enormous rate. When Miller wrote to his sister on October 5, he reported the camp had 10,000 cases and had

22 deaths that day. Unlike his previous account, this letter enumerated his symptoms. "I'll tell you how you feel when you have the flu," he wrote. The transcribed letter in the scrapbook presented the list exactly as below:

1. Severe pain in the head and temples throb.
2. Dizziness.
3. Pain in back from kidneys to shoulders.
4. Sore throat and a cold in lungs.
5. Sometimes sick in stomach.
6. Absolutely no ambition.[23]

The description echoed the accounts in the medical literature, including the accounts written by medical personnel at Camp Taylor. An article in the *Bulletin of the Johns Hopkins Hospital* described two types of symptoms, the first of which fit with Miller's: "constitutional reactions of an acute febrile disease—headache, general aching, chills, fever, malaise, prostration, anorexia, nausea or vomiting." The authors noted a second set of largely respiratory symptoms, and most likely those would have fit with Miller's once he entered the hospital with pneumonia.[24]

Despite his illness, Miller remained upbeat, believing that the worst was over. On October 6 he again wrote to his sister, opening his letter by observing "It is a beautiful morning." He then described the conditions in the camp "Adah, ambulances are running in every direction out here." He told her he was glad not to have reported his bout with the flu and observed, "They say you either get better or you get pneumonia very quickly." And added "I think by tomorrow I will be alright (sic)." Looking to the future as news of the war's likely conclusion was being reported he went on "I would like to see the war end but I would also like to get to France." It would be his last letter.[25]

The next day, Walton Fitzgerald, wrote to Miller's father to report that Miller had been hospitalized. Fitzgerald did his best to sound reassuring, claiming it was a preventive step taken for all suspicious cases, and that Miller had few symptoms. It is unclear whether Fitzgerald knew the real situation and was trying to sound upbeat or if he was unaware that Miller was gravely ill. He signed his letter "remember, there is no cause for worry!"[26]

An undated letter from the Acting Chaplain at Camp Taylor told a different story. He wrote to Miller's parents explaining that the young man was very sick with pneumonia. Although the medical staff provided everything for him, the Chaplain asked that his parents come to see him and he promised them "hope is not all gone. He has a fighting chance to pull through at present though he seems to have lost his nerve." He explained that the doctors and nurses were doing everything they could but that he needed "cheer." In many cases, parents rushed to military camps when their sons came down with influenza. An article in the *Indianapolis News* in October of 1918 about Camp Sherman in Ohio bore the headline "Mothers Go To Camp Despite Influenza." The government, it explained, provided relatives visiting hospitalized kin with masks and it paid for transportation back home for family members returning with the bodies for burial.[27]

Miller' parents did not make the trip to Louisville and they never saw him again. Three days after the Chaplain wrote to them, a telegram to the family arrived describing Miller as seriously ill. The next day another telegram reported his death. Some fellow soldiers, most likely hometown friends, wrote to the Miller family to offer condolences. The letter, sparked with patriotism and sympathy, said he "gave his life bravely for the great cause in which we are all united." The military appears to have sent his body home and 3 days after his death he was buried in Kingston. Corporal Miller had been in uniform and stateside for less than 3 months; the war ended a few weeks after his death.

Treating Influenza

A subsequent letter from Fitzgerald detailed the up-to-date medical treatments undertaken to save Miller' life. The information came by way of the unnamed nurse who attended him during his last days. Medical treatments, Fitzgerald learned from the nurse included blood transfusions and injections, neither of which provided any relief, but were done, he claimed, because "both doctors and nurses seemed to be gripped with the idea that 'Miller must not die.'" Given the vast number of cases and the enormous workload for nurses and physicians, this was probably a statement meant to provide comfort rather than an objective report about an individual case. The nursing sisters at Camp Taylor reportedly cared for between 120 and 150 men at a time and presumably the other nurses had a similar, overwhelming, patient load.[28]

In addition to efforts to provide symptomatic relief for pain and fever, physicians at Camp Taylor transfused into patients a serum produced from the blood of convalescent patients and another serum made from bacteria obtained from autopsy cultures and sensitized with the serum of recovered cases. In both cases donor patients were checked for a Wassermann reaction for syphilis. The goal of serum treatment was to boost resistance and it may well have done so in some cases. A recent review of the historical literature on the administration of convalescent serum in 1918 found several studies suggesting that individuals given serum had a reduced risk of death.[29]

For the most part, conditions in the overcrowded and understaffed military hospitals constrained effective use of serum therapy and prevented reliable studies of its value. Serums of different types were given and its administration could be haphazard or delayed to the point of being ineffective. Fitzgerald's letter refers to "injections"; it is not clear what kinds of injections Miller received or what they contained. The influenza literature refers to anal as well as subcutaneous injections and cites the application of various stimulants as well as morphine. The precise nature of the treatments Miller received, the conditions under which they were given, and their effects, if any, were not documented. Only his death and its aftermath received a full account in the family scrapbook.[30]

Religion and Medicine

Religious sentiments steeped in the promise of the hereafter infused many deathbed narratives before and after the influenza pandemic. In this vein, Fitzgerald wrote to Miller's father that that the young soldier was "conscious to the very end and died with his jaws set, well aware he was going to his Maker, but going without fear." It is difficult to believe that a nurse tending to up to 150 sick and dying patients at one time could have observed or known this. Most likely Miller's friend chose to provide words of comfort as he speculated about the final hours. He closed his letter by observing that the day would come when "united again in the Land of Rest, Miller can tell his Mother and Dad the things he wanted so much to say on his deathbed." The language was reminiscent of eighteenth and nineteenth century American accounts of death, particular with the mention of making peace with God, having a tranquil death, and of a future reunion in heaven. Similar religious sentiments appeared in a letter from a chaplain at Camp Funston, Kansas to a father in Missouri. His son, had "given his life in the Great Cause just as truly as any lad who falls on the battlefield of France," he wrote, reminding as well that the "Great God of the Universe and of men's souls is with us in our hours of trial."[31]

In the decades that followed the 1918 influenza pandemic the outbreak would take on new meanings, first as dramatic event not to be forgotten and later, in the late twentieth century, in the age of HIV/AIDS, and other infectious diseases, as a lesson in the limits of medical science and the need for preparing for future episodes. In the intervening years, however, medical science and public health became ever more effective and gained cultural authority. In the wake of these developments, deaths during disease outbreaks were increasingly recounted by patients and by families in medical as well as spiritual terms. The popular understanding of World War I and of the 1918 and 1919 influenza outbreaks would be uncoupled in the public imagination, even as medical historians carefully probed their links, paying attention to the experiences of communities on the home front and those sent to the battlefield. More recently, patients' memoirs of their illnesses have become a much more popular literary genre, while first hand accounts no longer reside family scrapbooks and collections of letters but increasingly live on patient websites and on other social media. The experiences of ordinary men and women, like Miller and others whose letters are described here, remain tucked away in archives, waiting to be reread because of the powerful testimony they hold about the lived experiences of life and death in the midst of an epidemic.

Acknowledgments

Thank you to Russell Johnson, Jennifer Gunn, Scott Podolsky, and Patricia D'Antonio for help with this manuscript.

Notes

1. Carol R. Byerly, "The U.S. Military and the Influenza Pandemics of 1918–1919," *Public Health Reports* 125 (2010): 82–91.

2. "Album of Photographs, Letters, Telegrams, and other Memorabilia Relating to the Brief Military Career, Illness, and Death by Pneumonia or Influenza of Alton William Miller of Kingston, New York, 1917–1918," Manuscript Collection no. 509.301, (hereafter Ms. Coll. no. 509.301) Special Collections, UCLA Louise M. Darling Biomedical Library (hereafter UCLA). See also, http://www.library.ucla.edu/events/influenza-pandemic-1918%E2%80%94-personal-narrative-heartbreaking-loss.   Other patient narratives can be found in Nancy K Bristow, "'It's as Bad as Anything Can Be': Patients, Identity, and the Influenza Pandemic," *Public Health Reports* 125 (2010): 134–44.

3. Alfred W. Crosby, *America's Forgotten Pandemic: The Influenza of 1918*, 2nd ed. (Cambridge: Cambridge University Press, 2003); John M. Barry, *The Great Influenza: The Story of the Deadliest Pandemic in History*, rev. ed. (New York: Penguin, 2005); Nancy K. Bristow, *American Pandemic: The Lost Worlds of the 1918 Influenza Epidemic*, reprint ed. (New York: Oxford University Press, 2017); Sandra Opdycke, *The Flu Epidemic of 1918: America's Experience in the Global Health Crisis* (New York: Routledge, 2014).

4. This analysis is drawn largely from the "Collection of personal narratives, manuscripts, and ephemera about the 1918–1919 influenza pandemic, 1917–1923," Collection 509, UCLA. Individual letters are identified by box and folder number or by collection number.

5. The lessons of the epidemic are discussed in Supplement 3, *Public Health Reports,* 125 (2010).

6. Letter from Alton W. Miller to Dear Adah, August 2, 1918, Camp Dix, New Jersey, Ms. Coll. no. 509.301, UCLA.

7. Carol R. Byerly, *Fever of War: The Influenza Epidemic in the U.S. Army during World War I* (New York: New York University Press, 2005), 75–76; and Opdycke page 48. The figure of 11,000 ill and 1,500 deaths comes from James C. Klotter, *Kentucky: Portrait in Paradox, 1900–1950* (Lexington: University of Kentucky Press, 1996), 239.

8. Autograph letter signed from Cyrus R. Lawrence, H.A. Barracks C-2, Naval Hospital, Pelham Bay Park, New York to his father, W.C. Lawrence, Columbus Ohio, October 24, 1918, Ms. Coll. no. 509.149, UCLA.

9. Letter from Alton W. Miller to Dear Adah, August 4, 1918, Camp Dix, New Jersey, Ms. Coll. No. 509.301, UCLA.

10. See, for example, Autograph letter signed from Arthur, 30th Field Artillery, Camp Funston, Kansas to his brother Fabian in Morgantown, Virginia, October 13, 1918, Ms. Coll. no. 509.106, UCLA.

11. Autograph letter signed from Hugh [Robertson?] aboard U.S.S. Don Juan de Austria at Newport, Rhode Island to Mrs. Anna Grace Robertson, Owensboro, Kentucky, October 5, 1918, Ms. Coll. no. 509.123, UCLA.

12. Typed letter signed from Midshipman first class G.T. "Jack" Huggins, U.S.S. Carola IV at Brest, France to his twin sister, Dollie, in St. Louis, Missouri, December 1918, Ms. Coll. no. 509.135, UCLA.

13. Autograph letter signed from Jesse E. Mooney, Kelly Field, San Antonio, Texas to Mrs. Chas [Charles] Mooney in Mantua, Portage County, Ohio, October 15, 1918, Ms. Coll. no. 509.182, UCLA.

14. Autograph letter signed from Private Wirden, Battery C, 36th Field Artillery Regiment, 12th Brigade, Camp McClellan, Alabama, to his mother, Mrs. A.E. Wirden, Fulton, New York, November 23, 1918, Ms. Coll. no. 509.114, UCLA.

15. Marnie McAllister, "Women Religious Came to the Army's Rescue in 1918," *Archdiocesan News*, July 13, 2016, https://therecordnewspaper.org/women-religious-came-armys-rescue-1918/; "More Nurses Are Needed at Camp Zachary Taylor: Women Urged to Volunteer," *Courier-Journal* (Louisville, Kentucky), October 7, 1918, https://www.newspapers.com/image/120033090. Accessed July 24, 2018.

16. Typed and autograph letter signed Carl [Carl D. Renne], France, to Dear sister Hazel [Miss Hazel M. Streifler], Pittsburgh, Pennsylvania, August 1, 1918. Ms. Coll. No. 509, Box 1 Folder 16, UCLA.

17. Letter from Albert to Dear Mother [Mrs. Mary Harbolt] Ironton, Ohio, October 6, 1918, Ms. Coll. no. 509, Box 1, Folder 24, UCLA.

18. Autograph letters signed Lambert, a cadet at U.S. Army Balloon School, Arcadia, California, to Mama, November 8, 1918, Ms. Coll. no. 509 Box 1 Folder 1, UCLA.

19. Letter from Walton W. Miller to Dear Father, October 5, 1918, Camp Taylor, Kentucky Ms. Coll. no. 509.301, UCLA.

20. Byerly, *Fever of War*, 85; and Dorothy A. Pettit and Janice Bailie, *A Cruel Wind: Pandemic Flu in America, 1918–1919* (Murfreesboro: Timberlane Books, 2008).

21. http://ocp.hul.harvard.edu/contagion/influenza.html Accessed July 24, 2018

22. *Kingston Daily Freeman*, October 23, 1918, 2, https://www.newspapers.com/image/28438522, and *Kingston Daily Freeman*, October 30, 1918, 2, https://www.newspapers.com/image/28439068. Accessed July 24, 2018

23. Letter from Alton W. Miller to Dear Adah, October 5, 1918, Camp Taylor, Kentucky, Ms. Coll. No. 509.301, UCLA.

24. "Proceedings of the Meeting of Camp and Base Surgeons, Camp Zachary Taylor, Kentucky, Thursday October 24, 1918," RG 112 Records of the Office of the Surgeon General, http://hdl.handle.net.2027/spo.6560flu.0014.656; and Arthur Bloomfield and George Harrop, Jr., "Clinical Observations on Epidemic Influenza," *Bulletin of the Johns Hopkins Hospital* 30 (January 1919): 1–9. Accessed July 24, 2018.

25. "The Influenzal Pandemic," *British Medical Journal* (July 13, 2018); and Letter from Alton W. Miller to Dear Adah, Camp Taylor, Kentucky, October 6, 1918 Ms. Coll. No. 509.301, UCLA. Accessed July 24, 2018

26. Letter from Walton G. Fitzgerald to Mr. Miller, Camp Taylor, Kentucky, October 7, 1918, Ms. Coll. no. 509.301, UCLA.

27. Letter from Gabriel Farrell, Acting Chaplin, Camp Taylor, Kentucky, undated probably October 7, 2018, Ms. Coll. No. 509.301; and "Mothers Go To Camp Despite Influenza," *Indianapolis News*, October 7, 1918, 5, https://www.newspapers.com/image/38409239.

28. McAllister, "Women Religious."

29. Office of the Surgeon General of the United States (Army) "Proceedings of the Meeting of Camp and Base Sugeons," 2; and "Medical and Scientific Conceptions of Influenza," https://virus.stanford.edu/uda/fluscimed.html; and Camp ZacharyTaylor, Kentucky T. C. Luke et al., "Meta-Analysis: Convalescent Blood Products for Spanish Influenza Pneumonia: A Future H5N1 Treatment?" *Annals of Internal Medicine* 154 (October 17, 2006): 599–609. October 24, 19198" RG 112 REcords of the Office of the Surgeon Genral https://quod.lib.umich.edu/cgi/t/text/idx/f/flu/6560flu.0014.656/1/–proceedings-of-the-meeting-of-camp-and-base-hospital?rgn=full+text;view=image;q1=Camp+Zachary+Taylor Accessed Oct 28, 2018.

30. Scott H. Podolsky, *Pneumonia Before Antibiotics: Therapeutic Evolution and Evaluation in Twentieth-Century America* (Baltimore: Johns Hopkins University Press, 2010), 9–50; Charles L. Mix, "Spanish Influenza in the Army," *New York Medical Journal* 108 (October 26, 1918): 709–18; "Epidemic Influenza," *JAMA* 71 (October 5, 1918): 1136–37; "The Influenzal Pandemic." The British Medical Journal 2, no. 3002 (1918): 39. http://www.jstor.org.proxy.libraries.rutgers.edu/stable/20310518 Accessed December 12, 2018Preston Kyes, "The Treatment of Lobar Pneumonia with an Anti-Pneumococcous Serum," *Journal of Medical Research* 38 (July 1918): 495–501.

31. Letter from Frank W. Herriott to A.J. Little, October 10, 1918, in Collection of letters and documents about the military service and death by influenza and pneumonia of Private Charles M.P. Little of Dunnegan, Missouri, at Headquarters Company, 29th Field Artillery, 10th Division, U.S. Army, Camp Funston, Fort Riley, Kansas, Ms. Coll. no. 509.100, UCLA.

Disclosure. The author has no relevant financial interest or affiliations with any commercial interests related to the subjects discussed within this article.

JANET GOLDEN, PhD
Professor of History
Rutgers University–Camden

MEDIA REVIEWS

Power to Heal: Medicare and the Civil Rights Revolution. 2018. Producers: Barbara Berney, Roberta Friedman, and Daniel Loewenthal; Directors: Charles Burnett and Daniel Loewenthal. BLB Film Productions. www.blbfilmproductions.com

Power to Heal: Medicare and the Civil Rights Revolution uses the history of race and health policy to illustrate how black medical and civil rights leaders, grass roots activists, and the federal government worked together to desegregate America's hospitals, and secure more equitable and accessible healthcare for black Americans. The film expands the narrative of the civil rights movement beyond a fight for voting privileges, jobs, education, and housing to include a lesser known battle—the eradication of a racially separate and unequal healthcare system.

Power to Heal employs an impressive range of primary sources, including oral histories with nurses and community members, photographs, and archival data to advance the argument that Medicare legislation desegregated our nation's hospitals. With the passage of the Civil Rights Act of 1964 and the Social Security Amendments Act of 1965, which created Medicare and Medicaid, the federal government had both a legislative mandate to guarantee all citizens equal access to hospitals that received federal funds, and a universal insurance program to enforce it. Simply put, hospitals that did not comply with Title VI of the Civil Rights Act which "forbade discrimination on the basis of race, color, and national origin" would be denied Medicare reimbursement.[1] In dramatic style, viewers experience the frantic push by President Lyndon B. Johnson's administration to successfully integrate thousands of hospitals in just 3 months, and in the process, avert a national crisis that would have left countless Medicare beneficiaries without access to medical care.

The diversity in authoritative voice is a key strength of the film that helps move the narrative beyond the stereotypical depiction of black Americans as merely powerless victims of Jim Crow racism and neglect, and highlights the racial uplift that was occurring within the black community prior to federal intervention. As the film demonstrates, black physicians established and operated hospitals and nursing schools across the nation in response to segregation and institutionalized racism that locked them out of mainstream institutions.

Nursing History Review 28 (2020): 196–198. A Publication of the American Association for the History of Nursing. Copyright © 2020 Springer Publishing Company.
http://dx.doi.org/10.1891/1062-8061.28.196

It was also black medical and civil rights leaders who led the landmark *Simkins v Moses H. Cone Memorial Hospital* civil suit that successfully challenged the "separate but equal" clause of the Hill Burton Act of 1946, a program that provided federal funding for construction and improvement of hospitals.

The strengths of this film are many, but some underlying weaknesses are worth examining. In presenting the dramatic push to integrate hospitals, the filmmakers gloss over the thousands of *white Americans* who were also at risk if hospitals did not desegregate. The Johnson administration's novel strategy was in making healthcare access, which was largely viewed and experienced as a "black problem," a serious concern for white America. Though Johnson's plan was politically savvy and highly effective, its premise rested on, and inherently upheld, white supremacy ideology. A critical analysis of how race (versus racism) has been instituted and reinforced, as both a political and biological category in law and health policy to suppress and enforce universal healthcare rights would have added much-needed depth to the film.

Also, the extraordinary organizing work of black nurses is missing from this story of hospital desegregation. The nurses' activism is essential to this history, since it was their work that inspired the later movement toward a fully integrated healthcare system.[2] For example military hospitals broke the color line in 1945 after the National Association of Colored Graduate Nurses, a separate organization established by black nurses in 1908, led a successful movement to desegregate and integrate the United States armed forces during World War II.[3] Black nurses took advantage of this victory and the war-induced nursing shortage and began integrating civilian hospitals, nursing schools, and state associations in the early post-war years, and by 1965 many hospitals, particularly in the north and west, were already desegregated.[4] In a sense, the film's core argument is qualified by the primary sources presented, however, a more expansive search of the archives and historiographical literature would have revealed these important omissions.

Narrated by award-winning actor Danny Glover, *Power to Heal* brings to light a moving account of how our nation's hospitals were transformed from racially separate and unequal institutions into a more integrated system. Only 56 minutes in length, the documentary serves as a nice entry point into the history of segregated healthcare. Those seeking a deeper understanding of this history will need to seek out additional sources. The film will appeal to a wide audience, but it is ideal for health professionals, policy makers, and scholars who can provide deeper insight about the history of race and American healthcare. It would be especially useful to undergraduate and graduate curriculums in nursing and medical education, the medical humanities, Africana studies, and public health.

Race and racism is deeply rooted in our nation's healthcare system. Considering the recent initiatives to repeal and/or reform the Affordable Care Act, *Power to Heal* is both timely and highly significant to our current healthcare context, and contributes to the growing body of historical knowledge about our nation's racial past.[5]

Notes

1. The United States Department of Justice, "Overview of Title VI of the Civil Rights Act of 1964," accessed January 10, 2018, https://www.justice.gov/crt/fcs/TitleVI-Overview.

2. Mary Elizabeth Carnegie, *The Path We Tread: Blacks in Nursing, 1854–1984* (Philadelphia: Lippincott, 1986); Darlene Clark Hine, *Black Women in White: Racial Conflict and Cooperation in the Nursing Profession, 1890–1950* (Bloomington: Indiana University Press, 1989), 102; Darlene Clark Hine, "Mabel Keaton Staupers: The integration of black nurses into the Armed Forces, World War II," in *Black Leaders of the Twentieth Century* (Madison, WI: University of Wisconsin Press, 1984).

3. Hine, *Black Women in White*; Charissa Threat, *Nursing Civil Rights: Gender and Race in the Army Nurse Corps* (Chicago: University of Illinois Press, 2015).

4. David McBride, *Integrating the City of Medicine* (Philadelphia: Temple University Press, 1989).

5. Frank J. Thompson, Michael K. Gusmano, and Shugo Shinohara, "Trump and the Affordable Care Act: Congressional Repeal Efforts, Executive Federalism, and Program Durability," *Publius: The Journal of Federalism* 48, no. 3 (2018): 396–424; Julie Rovner and Kaiser Health News, "Timeline: Despite GOP's Failure To Repeal Obamacare, The ACA Has Changed," *The Washington Post*, April 5, 2018; Kate Zernike, Reed Abelson, and Abby Goodnough, "New Effort to Kill Obamacare Is Called 'the Most Radical'," *The New York Times*, September 21, 2017.

Hafeeza Anchrum, MSN, RN
University of Pennsylvania School of Nursing
418 Curie Blvd
Philadelphia, PA 19104

The History of the FDA's Fight for Consumer Protection and Public Health.
U.S. Food and Drug Administration, Silver Springs, MD.
(https://www.fda.gov/AboutFDA/History/default.htm)

The United States Food and Drug Administration (FDA) website "The History
of the FDA's Fight for Consumer Protection and Public Health," follows the
changing scale and scope of the agency from its roots in agricultural chemical
testing in the late 1840s, through the vast expansion of regulatory powers from
the 1938 Federal Food, Drug, and Cosmetic Act, to the many roles it plays
today. The site contains a trove of primary and secondary source materials;
photographs, videos, oral histories, legal documents, digitized exhibits, and
essays demonstrate the agency's long-term focus on consumer protection and
public health.

The shining star of this website is its collection of historical images, which
contains over 250 images of artifacts, ephemera, photographs, and other materials from the agency's archives. Housed on the online photo management and
sharing platform Flickr, the *FDA History* photo album provides snapshots into
the products, events, people, and policies that have shaped the agency's development.[1] The high quality images and detailed captions allow the collection to
reach professional and amateur historians, educators, and students alike. The
historical context and depth provided in the image descriptions are an exciting
introduction for undergraduate or graduate students to the history of public
health, consumer protection, and U.S. government regulations.

Videos from the FDA's archives are another an important component of
a series of videos on the FDA site. The *From the FDA Vault* videos highlight
products and materials the agency has sought to remove from the market, as
well as tools and technologies that have contributed to the surveillance of consumer products. These short, digestible clips emphasize the successes, failures,
and limitations of the FDA as a regulatory body, and work well as an intro-
ductory device for anyone unfamiliar with the agency's history and mission.[2]

In addition to media content, the FDA site contains links to a variety
of primary source texts of interest to consumers and researchers. The press
releases, warning letters, and consumer updates are more current in nature,
and they will be most useful to researchers or other individuals interested in
the agency's modern history. Older primary source materials are listed. These
materials span a broader range of time and subject, and the site provides links to
their holding institutions. The link for FDA Notices of Judgments from 1908

Nursing History Review 28 (2020): 199–202. A Publication of the American Association for the History
of Nursing. Copyright © 2020 Springer Publishing Company.
http://dx.doi.org/10.1891/1062-8061.28.199

to 1964, for example, leads to a digital database maintained by the National Library of Medicine.[3]

The Notices of Judgments are a particularly interesting component of this collection. The notices are short summaries of court cases against violative products that provide a window into ongoing and episodic issues the FDA faced through much of the 20th century. Prophylactics riddled with holes and canned veggies contaminated with bug parts were, for instance, a repeating area of concern.[4] While the sale of amphetamine sulfate tablets without a prescription—often at truck stops and gas stations—was a problem apparently confined to the early 1950s and 1960s.[5] The patterns and trends revealed by FDA judgments lead naturally to a wide variety of historical questions—how were prophylactics manufactured throughout the 20th century? did manufacturing methods contribute to product failure or food contamination? why was there a spike in cases against amphetamine distributors? why were amphetamines so popular at gas stations? were FDA interventions effective?—such possibilities make this collection a particularly great resource for history educators in search of strong starting points for research-based assignments for undergraduate or graduate students.

Another valuable set of primary sources on the FDA site are transcripts of interviews conducted through the FDA's Oral History program, which began in the late 1970s.[6] Designed to supplement and also distill the physical collections pertaining to the history of the agency, the program has captured the voices of employees who worked at all levels, in a variety of different positions, and across geographic locations at the FDA. Interviews with directors of various divisions and bureaus, regulatory review and consumer safety officers, chemists, microbiologists, veterinarians, and lawyers, provide fascinating snapshots into the agency's past.

Despite interesting and engaging content, the FDA's history website can be confusing and user-hostile. The homepage, for example, has navigation systems that don't align with one another, and have links that connect to different pages, with similar content. This, combined with omnipresent broken links, makes it very difficult to follow where materials are located within the site. Functionality is further complicated by the site's reliance on Archive-It, a web archiving service that captures and preserves online content.[7] For instance, in order to find the oral history collection users must make their way through the current site and then through the site as it was designed when captured by Archive-It. These additional layers make it even more challenging to access and use the sources on the site.

Despite the frustrating and time-consuming experience of navigating the FDA's history website, professional historians, dedicated researchers, and faculty teaching classes focused on U.S. policy or regulatory affairs, consumer protection, public health, and/or medical and nutritional history may find the effort worthwhile, as the site has several valuable primary source collections. The casual consumer, however, may be better off accessing the historical content on more user-friendly platforms such as the FDA Flickr account, FDA YouTube channel—even the FDA's Twitter, @US_FDA.[8]

Notes

1. The *FDA History* photo album, found at https://www.flickr.com/photos/fdaphotos/albums/72157624615595535, is one of many interesting albums within the "U.S. Food and Drug Administration" Flickr page, found at https://www.flickr.com/photos/fdaphotos/.

2. The *From the Vault* videos are also available on YouTube, found at https://www.youtube.com/playlist?list=PLey4Qe-UxcxasCYYH4p-P8kIyMqah386U. A playlist within the "U.S. Food and Drug Admin" YouTube channel, found at https://www.youtube.com/channel/UC_giJ3xlEL9jUF1YfJdzzuQ.

3. The FDA Notices of Judgment collection is available on the National Library of Medicine's site found at https://fdanj.nlm.nih.gov/

4. *U.S. v. 2 1/16 Gross of Prophylactic,* No. 29279 (W. Dist. New York, December, 1938), FDA Notices of Judgment, https://fdanj.nlm.nih.gov/catalog/fdnj29279; *U.S. v. 19 Packages and 40 ½ Gross of Prophylactics,* No. 3125 (W. Dist. of Missouri, November, 1945), FDA Notices of Judgment, https://fdanj.nlm.nih.gov/catalog/ddnj01325; *U.S. v. 175 Gross,* No. 3734 (Dist. of Colorado, November, 1952), FDA Notices of Judgment, https://fdanj.nlm.nih.gov/catalog/ddnj03734; *U.S. v. 1,000 Cans of Tomato Pulp,* No. 4295 (Dist. of New Jersey, June, 1916) FDA Notices of Judgment, https://fdanj.nlm.nih.gov/catalog/fdnj04295; *S. Dist. Miss. v. Oconomowoe Canning Co.,* No. 27210 (S. Dist. of Missouri, August, 1961) FDA Notices of Judgemnt, https://fdanj.nlm.nih.gov/catalog/ffnj27210.

5. *U.S. v. Hy-Gold Drug Co., Inc., and Boris Golden,* No. 3948 (N. Dist. of Illinois, August, 1953), FDA Notices of Judgment, https://fdanj.nlm.nih.gov/catalog/ddnj03948; *S. Dist. Ind. v. William Albert Bork, t/a Bork's Truck Stop,* No. 6125 (S. D. of Indiana, December, 1960), FDA Notices of Judgment, https://fdanj.nlm.nih.gov/catalog/ddnj06125; *Northern District of Georgia v. Charles Frank Gray, t/a Charles' Truck Stop,* No. 6245 (N. Dist. of Georgia, March, 1961), FDA Notices of Judgment, https://fdanj.nlm.nih.gov/catalog/ddnj06245

6. Transcripts of some interviews are available through the FDA's site, while tapes (and sometimes transcripts) are available in person at the History of Medicine Division of the National Library of Medicine.

7. The FDA's reliance on Archive-It also raises a (small) red flag about their commitment to updating and maintaining historical content on their site. Archive-It is a product of Internet Archive, a non-profit public digital library that aims to permanently store and maintain digital content. Both are trusted and reliable services, but it is nonetheless concerning that valuable materials such as oral histories are *not* hosted on the current site and are only available through the archived website. See https://archive-it.org/ and https://archive.org/about/ to learn more about these services.

8. Most of the content on Twitter reflects current or of-the-moment issues. Occasionally the "U.S. FDA" account posts information related to the history of the agency. Such posts are identified (and thus can be search using) with the hash-tag *#FDAHistory.* The "U.S. FDA" account can be found at https://twitter.com/US_FDA?ref_src=twsrc%5Egoogle%7Ctwcamp%5Eserp%7Ctwgr%5Eauthor

Disclosure. The author has no relevant financial interest or affiliations with any commercial interests related to the subjects discussed within this article.

ELIZABETH SEMLER
PhD Candidate
Program in the History of Science, Technology, and Medicine
University of Minnesota
May Building (MMC 506)
420 Delaware St. SE,
Minneapolis, MN 55455

All My Babies: A Midwife's Own Story. 1952. Georgia Department of Public Health, Medical Audio-Visual Institute of the Association of American Medical Colleges. Producer: George C. Stoney; Director: George C. Stoney. ($19.95, Amazon.com. Also available at https://www.youtube.com/watch?v=I2djFnp 5h0w)

Education for Childbirth: Labor & Childbirth. 1950. Medical Films, Inc. Producer: Photo & Sound Productions, San Francisco; Director: D. M. Hatfield. (https://www.youtube.com/watch?v=7Bwmv4fenDo)

High maternal and infant mortality rates in the United States in the early 20th century placed maternity care at the forefront of social reform efforts. Subsequent improvements in childbirth outcomes were slow in Southeastern states particularly among rural African American women. Traditional black midwives, who attended the majority of births in rural American Southern communities, were blamed for the high rates of maternal and infant mortality. The two films, *All My Babies: A Midwife's Own Story* and *Education for Childbirth: Labor and Childbirth*, feature Southern communities, and reflect the changes that were taking place worldwide as hospitals and physicians became central in a previously midwife-led, home-based experience.

The 1951 teaching film *All My Babies* covers 118 teaching points for traditional black midwives, through the example and work of Mary Coley, an experienced black midwife who attended births in rural Albany, Georgia from the 1930s to the 1960s. Conversely, *Education for Childbirth: Labor and Childbirth* was produced in 1950 to provide education for expectant women, typically white, planning to give birth in the hospital. Together these films highlight the changes in maternity care that took place in the United States in the mid-20th century: moving from midwives to physicians, from home to hospital, and from a focus on the mother and her labor to the physician and his work.

Filmmaker George Stoney wrote, directed, and produced *All my babies* for the Georgia Department of Public Health. Coley cares for two women, Ida and Marybelle, during pregnancy, labor, and birth.[1] Coley narrates the film, explaining the procedures mothers can expect at the health department's prenatal visits, and pointing out preparations needed prior to childbirth. Coley's midwifery care is shown throughout Ida's labor and the birth of "another little old healthy boy." A beautiful birth sequence shows the mother's face, the midwife's work, and the birth of the infant, and ends with mother and

Nursing History Review 28 (2020): 203–206. A Publication of the American Association for the History of Nursing. Copyright © 2020 Springer Publishing Company.
http://dx.doi.org/10.1891/1062-8061.28.203

baby together in bed, Coley at the bedside assisting with breastfeeding. Ida's experience contrasts sharply with Marybelle's who failed to complete all the preparations recommended by health department officials. Her son is born prematurely, requiring an incubator. Marybelle's poor nutrition and lack of preparation are blamed for the less than optimal outcome.

The film's purpose as a training tool for midwives is achieved as Coley methodically reviews the teaching points identified by supervising nurse-midwives Hannah Mitchell and Marian Cadwallader, both white. A discussion of screening for pregnancy complications, testing for syphilis, and the importance of good nutrition provide foundational knowledge of prenatal care for the midwives. The lack of cleanliness is identified as a major problem among the midwives as demonstrated during a midwife class at the health department. A physician lectures the midwives about an infant who died "that oughtn't to have" due to an infected cord. The physician's assertion is that something wasn't clean. Whether it was scissors, dressing, or hands that weren't clean, the midwife was to blame. Racial, gendered, and class biases of the era are demonstrated as the white male physician stands over the black female midwives, chastising them for their failures. The film then outlines strategies for addressing these failures.

Filmed in Dougherty County homes, *All My Babies* provides a glimpse of the harsh realities of life in the 1950s in the rural Southeastern United States. An inside look of Coley's and Ida's homes reveals modest but comfortable residences that meet the needs of the families inhabiting them. However, the shack where Marybelle's birth takes is small, minimally furnished, drafty, and untidy. These contrasting settings demonstrated the necessity of cleanliness and preparation for childbirth for the midwives of the time. For today's audience, they vividly highlight how access to basic resources impacted health and explained health disparities of the time.

The musical score of *All My Babies* adds to the interest and significance of the documentary. Acapella singing by The Musical Art Chorus of Washington D. C. provides background music for the film. Lyrics of black spiritual hymns were rewritten to reflect childbirth and aspects of the film such as "Everything's ready for the baby." This musical device feels overdone at first listen but works in the end. The harmonies of the amateur choir set the stage for training the midwives, drawing them in with familiar melodies.

All My Babies offers unique film documentation of the work of 20th-century midwives in the Southeastern US, including many of the racial and cultural insensitivities that midwives and their clients would encounter. The film captures and preserves Coley's work providing woman-centered maternity care and supporting physiologic birth. The film is a classic in midwifery history and was selected for the National Film Registry by the Library of Congress for being "culturally, historically or aesthetically significant."

The *Education for Childbirth* film of the same era preserves a very different historical phenomenon. It follows the labor and birth of an unnamed woman. A male narrator reviews items that should be packed in preparation for a hospital birth including "things to make you pretty." The course of labor and birth is described, and information guiding when the mother should proceed to the hospital is given. The narrator reassures the mother that the doctor will arrive soon after she does "and take charge." Expectant mothers viewing the film in 1950 were encouraged to relinquish all control to the physician. Choices for anesthesia are presented, but the mother is asked to "by all means, leave the decision in your doctor's hands."

The birth scene in this short educational film is markedly different from those in *All My Babies*. In *Childbirth Education*, the camera focuses on the physician throughout the birth, never showing the mother's face. The infant is glimpsed as the physician completes his work and presents the mother with a view of her clean baby. New parents are instructed to prepare birth announcements, call relatives, and buy cigars and candy to distribute among well-wishers. The take-home message for viewers is "you can rely on your doctor and his helpers."

Viewing these films offers today's audiences a glimpse into some of the last vestiges of the old ways and insight into the historical context of the new approach to childbirth. The films portray the complicity of the nursing and medical professions in the elimination of traditional healers and midwives during the 20th century, providing valuable lessons for nursing and medical students. The films are first-hand records of the history of childbirth in the United States for American History education courses. Historians, midwives, physicians, nurses, medical anthropologists, students of women's studies, and those interested in the history of childbirth would benefit from the story told in these films.

Notes

1. Mary Coley lined up about six pregnant women under her care to be in the film, though most of them gave birth before the filming began. Martha Sapp was chosen, and given the pseudonym Ida. Sapp was compensated for the cost of her delivery, clothing, supplies, baby sitters, travel expenses, and a new refrigerator. Marybelle, the second woman whose birth is shown, portrayed a very different role than she lived, representing a woman giving birth in squalid condition. In her own life she was a student at Albany College and her husband, who is also in the film, was a Sergeant at a local airfield. There is no information available about what kind of compensation she received, or whether Marybelle

was a pseudonym. L. Jackson, "The Production of George Stoney's Film All My Babies: A Midwife's Own Story (1952)," *Film History* 1 (1987): 367–92.

Disclosure. The author has no relevant financial interest or affiliations with any commercial interests related to the subjects discussed within this article.

Eileen J. B. Thrower, CNM, PhD, APRN
Frontier Nursing University
195 School St.
Hyden, KY 41749

BOOK REVIEWS

Florence Nightingale, Nursing, and Healthcare Today
By Lynn McDonald
(New York: Springer Publishing Company, 2017) (256 pages; $55.00 paperback)

As the bicentenary of Florence Nightingale's birth approaches in May 2020, this is a timely addition to the works on her life and legacy. Often described as the world's most famous nurse, the breadth and depth of Nightingale's work and ideas are not always appreciated by a modern audience and she been the subject of a sometimes hostile press in recent years.

Lynn McDonald is well placed to challenge some of the misconceptions that exist about her as a pre-eminent Nightingale scholar and well published author in this field, including her work as editor of the sixteen volumes of her collected works. Drawing on in depth knowledge of Nightingale's work (which is, McDonald points out, far wider than her best known "Notes on Nursing") she argues that her book is "geared to telling a story that has often been missed or botched by the use of poor secondary sources."

The first part of the book is divided into chapters, each of which deals with what, she terms, the "core concepts" of Nightingale's work, which include health promotion, ethics, infection control, paediatric nursing, long-term and palliative care, administration and research policy, and advocacy. These, she argues "have transcended time to influence nursing today" and she illustrates in a lively and accessible way the impact of Nightingale's work and how it still resonates today. Each chapter ends with some helpful "questions for discussion."

The second section of the book features excerpts from some of Nightingale's work including some of her less well-known later writings, in which McDonald demonstrates how some of her earlier ideas evolved alongside advances in science. Thus, Nightingale's often quoted denial of germ theory (preferring instead it is argued to espouse miasma theory based upon the concept that it is the smell that causes the disease) is shown by McDonald to have changed over time and she was thus far from refuting germ theory.

Nursing History Review 28 (2020): 207–208. A Publication of the American Association for the History of Nursing. Copyright © 2020 Springer Publishing Company.
http://dx.doi.org/10.1891/1062-8061.28.207

There is also a very useful appendix, which features a detailed timeline of Nightingale's work and legacy.

A few aspects of the book did jar with me. She is understandably frustrated with commentators whom she feels have misrepresented Nightingale and her ideas in an often hostile way. She refutes their claims in some details in the book and points to the many errors which she has discerned in their writings. At times though, this discourse did seem to dominate the narrative and feels strident in tone.

McDonald also does make some sweeping statements, for example when she discusses nursing before Nightingale the classic stereotyped image is presented unquestioningly and is not referenced. "The women called 'nurses' before her reforms, apart from those in religious orders," she states "were low paid, disreputable and often drunk," a view which has been challenged by more nuanced discussions of the origins of modern nursing.

Throughout the book, though, McDonald's knowledge of Nightingale's work shines through and she has done an admirable job in presenting the breadth and depth of Nightingale's work, and how it is still resonates today for a modern audience, in a succinct and erudite way. It is a useful addition to the plethora of writing about Nightingale. Its scholarship, size, and reasonable price will make this an attractive purchase for those wanting to reflect on Nightingale's work and impact.

CLAIRE CHATTERTON
Staff Tutor
School of Health, Wellbeing and Social Care
The Open University
Milton Keynes
MK7 6AA
England

A Time of Scandal: Charles R. Forbes, Warren G. Harding, and the Making of the Veterans Bureau

By Rosemary Stevens

(Baltimore, MD: Johns Hopkins University Press, 2016) (376 pages; $34.95 cloth)

The latest book from Rosemary Stevens, a distinguished scholar of the history of public health, medicine, and health policy, is an epic tale of scandal. Depicting the brief tenure and disastrous downfall of Charles Forbes, the post-World War I director of the federal agency now known as the Department of Veterans Affairs, it accomplishes at least three feats. First, it calls into question a century-old historiographical truism: Forbes was a crook. Second, it compels the reader to ponder why political scandals erupt, what they accomplish, and the damage they leave in their wakes. Finally, Stevens' picture of 1920s Washington, which includes vivid details of marriages, love affairs, and family dynamics, demonstrates that public and private life are inextricably—sometimes perilously—linked.

Drawing from an array of archives, as well as newly unearthed personal collections of Forbes' descendants, Stevens shows that her central character's early career was shaped by his immigrant parents and working class roots, his professional experience as a construction planner and manager, and his friendships—especially one with Warren G. Harding. When Harding became president in 1921, he prioritized finding positions in his administration for associates, including Forbes, who was assigned the massive task of overseeing veterans' health, insurance, and vocational education benefits at the Bureau of War Risk Insurance, which would soon become the Veterans' Bureau.

Forbes entered the position, Stevens notes, determined to succeed in the face of considerable challenges. His predecessor reportedly told him, ". . . you are coming into a job that will bring you only grief and sorrow" (p. 52). But Forbes worked "nonstop," Stevens says, with a "sense of mission" (pp. 82–83). At a moment when veterans' groups were demanding that comprehensive services be made available immediately, he urgently pursued an expansive hospital-building program. In the process, he was, as Stevens puts it, "stacking up a pile of influential foes" (p. 98), who were concerned and suspicious about his lack of cost-consciousness.

Nursing History Review 28 (2020): 209–211. A Publication of the American Association for the History of Nursing. Copyright © 2020 Springer Publishing Company.
http://dx.doi.org/10.1891/1062-8061.28.209

Gradually, as Forbes was held responsible for problems big and small in an unwieldy system, he eventually came to believe that "the Veterans' Bureau was 'the biggest lemon ever given to an hombre to run'" (p. 145). As a case in point, Stevens points out, "it was not Forbes' fault that New York lacked hospital beds . . . but who else was there to blame?" (p. 137) Stevens notes that correspondence between Harding and Forbes is missing from the archival record, but she pieces together clues indicating that the president's confidence in his Bureau director was eroding. Exhausted, physically ailing, and on the verge of divorce from his wife, Forbes resigned from his post in 1923.

Soon after, a bipartisan Senate investigation shifted its focus from a problem-laden Veterans' Bureau to Forbes' individual actions, Stevens argues, not because there was hard evidence of illegal behavior, but because of political motive. Senators—"self-righteous men [who] howled for revenge" (p. 225)—went after the former director with the aim of appearing as saviors of military veterans. For Republicans, bringing down Forbes protected the party's image by contributing to a larger narrative that pegged Harding not as a lackluster leader, but as a victim of greedy and foolish friends.

The linchpin of the government's case against Forbes, Stevens maintains, was the testimony of Elias Mortimer. "One of a crowd of lobbyists, publicists, and fixers who descended on Washington during the wartime boom," Mortimer made a career of ensnaring public figures in shady activities, then bringing them down (p. 101); a congressman who had fallen victim to his schemes described him as a "paragon of mendacity" (p. 105). Mortimer accompanied Forbes on official Veterans' Bureau trips, where he introduced him to construction industry insiders and helped ensure access to liquor and festivities. In government hearings, Forbes testified that there was nothing untoward about these interactions. Mortimer, who suspected that his wife and the gregarious bureaucrat were having an affair, signed on as a protected government witness and maintained that he and Forbes were, in fact, working together to steal federal funds.

Multiple witnesses cast doubt on Mortimer's portrayal of Forbes as a classless swindler, Stevens notes, but just enough circumstantial evidence existed to make the allegations believable. In the eyes of a "tribunal" of Senate investigators, Forbes was an outsider with a questionable pedigree (p. 190). He had aggressively built a health program while flagrantly disregarding expense. And he was irresponsible in private life, too: while working as a civil servant, he had purchased a showy new car and cavorted with women at raucous parties. Those activities, along with the fact that Mortimer said what the press and public "wanted to hear" sealed the case against Forbes (p. 307). He was found guilty of conspiracy, and sent to the federal penitentiary at Leavenworth for a two-year sentence.

Using archival sleuthing, Stevens shows that the scandal resonated in the lives of Forbes, who avoided the public eye until his death in 1952, and his family members. It also lived on in the historical record. Like newspaper reports of the 1920s, accounts of Forbes published throughout the last century have recounted his illicit behaviors and taken his guilt as proven fact.

Stevens' study challenges the reader to question narratives of good and evil, and to consider distinctions between imperfect behavior and criminal malevolence. Worthwhile and engaging reading for scholars of the interwar years, bureaucracies, and American political development, it shows that scandals, which have the potential to entertain and satisfy many and harm relatively few, may be an attractive, but somewhat ineffectual way to solve complex political problems.

JESSICA L. ADLER
Assistant Professor of History and Health Policy & Management
Florida International University

Irish Medical Education and Student Culture, c.1850–1950
By Laura Kelly

(Liverpool, UK: Liverpool University Press, 2011) (276 pages; $120.00; hardcover)

In contrast to the noticeably whiggish character of earlier monograph histories of modern scientific medicine in Ireland, Irish medical historiography in the twenty-first century offers a more critical scholarship, due in much part, to its location within medical humanities departments and academic centers in Ireland, the UK and elsewhere. Laura Kelly's *Irish Medical Education and Student Culture, c.1850–1950* represents a valuable addition to contemporary analytical and contextual medical historiography and addresses a topic that, somewhat surprisingly, has not been treated to the same extent as, for example, the history of nursing education. The book comprehensively describes and analyses the development of medical education, with a particular focus on the profiles, curricular experiences, training culture and the social life of the medical student. Presented in seven chapters, the book covers a century of developments, beginning in 1850, when Irish medicine had established an international reputation for its treatment methods and scientific discoveries and apprenticeship training was replaced by a standardized curriculum, and ending in 1950, when women had established their place in medical schools.

Kelly examines how the medical pupils' image and role expectations over the latter half of the nineteenth century were transformed from one of potentially corruptible young men to heroes engaged in a "manly and noble profession." The association of medicine with "manliness and masculinity" became part of the prevailing discourse and may account for the common usage of the moniker "medical man" in normative texts and in wider professional discourse.

Kelly discusses the class background of medical students and writes that "social mobility and a sense of middle-class respectability" were part of the motivation for pursuing medical education. She identifies the various feeder secondary schools that provided applicants to the medical schools and highlights the factors that influenced a student's choice of medical school, which included a school's reputation and students' personal preferences, such as convenience of location, availability of sporting opportunities, and the level of fees. The medical students' social and religious backgrounds are further illustrated with detailed summary tables, demonstrating that students were drawn from commercial-merchant, agricultural-industrial, and professional classes,

Nursing History Review 28 (2020): 212–214. A Publication of the American Association for the History of Nursing. Copyright © 2020 Springer Publishing Company.
http://dx.doi.org/10.1891/1062-8061.28.212

including medicine, law and the clergy. Religious affiliation and social class in combination also determined the profile of the student; hence, for example, the student at Trinity College Dublin was largely upper-middle class and Protestant.

A major theme in the book is the student's training experience, which in the "pre-clinical years" included lectures in the basic sciences, instruction in the laboratory and dissecting room and clinical instruction in the hospital, where for most students, "real" medical training began. Extra-curricular activities included sports and membership of biological and medical student societies, which served important social and professionalization functions. Kelly also examines rites of passage, such as the transition from "gyb"—the "boyish" first-year student—to the fully formed mature "medicus," who had endured pre-clinical studies, clinical training and the hardships and deprivations of student life. The author discusses how these rites of passage occurred in spaces like the lecture theatre, the dissecting room and the sports field and became "imbued with masculine tropes." The boisterousness and mischief making in the lecture theatre, emotional detachment and strength of nerve in the dissecting room, and competitiveness in the sports field were all expressions of masculinity that rendered the training school as a space where hegemonic masculinity was fostered and expressed. In these spaces, the female medical student—"the lady medical"—was largely a spectator.

Kelly dedicates an entire chapter to women in Irish medical schools and places women's admission into medical schools within the wider context of women in higher education in the Victorian period. She argues that, while prospective women doctors experienced the same opposition and prejudice to women in higher education as their counterparts in other fields of education, the medical hierarchy was more open-minded when it came to admitting women. Nevertheless, in medical education discourses, prevailing ideas that higher education could result in a loss of womanliness were common, and while "lady medicals" were portrayed as studious and hardworking, they were also subjected to sexual objectification and ridicule by their male counterparts. Women in medical schools were cast as a separate part of the student body; as "others," they experienced separate instruction in the dissecting room and socialized in separate spaces, like college "ladies rooms."

The last part of the book examines the training experience of medical students in the period 1920–1950, and the narrative is informed by oral history interviews, which the author conducted. These testimonies reference classroom and clinical experiences, social life, and career opportunities, and the continuing treatment of women as a separate part of the student body. Testimonies also reference the image of the medical student, which somewhat counteract the myth of the student as "boisterous and rowdy."

The chapters are structured chronologically and thematically and the narrative is brisk and engaging. Each chapter is closed with helpful conclusions, which draw together the author's principal arguments. As evidenced in the extensive footnotes and bibliography, the book is thoroughly researched and the narrative is informed by a judicious mix of both primary and secondary sources, including documentary sources, matriculation registers, student magazines and periodicals, individual memoirs, and oral testimonies. As with much Irish social history, themes of social class, gender, and sectarian tensions recur, and these themes are expertly weaved throughout the narrative. Kelly concludes that by presenting a "bottom-up" view of the history of medical education in Ireland, the book offers a different methodological approach to the more traditional focus on university staff, and in so doing, reinstates the voices of the students themselves. This claim is well justified in this comprehensive, well-written and scholarly social history of Irish medical schools.

GERARD M. FEALY
Professor of Nursing, Dean of Nursing and Head of School
UCD School of Nursing, Midwifery and Health Systems
University College Dublin
Ireland

Lady Lushes: Gender, Alcoholism, and Medicine in Modern History

By Michelle McClellan

(New Brunswick, NJ: Rutgers University Press, 2017) (237 pages; $39.95 paperback)

Michelle McClellan's *Lush Ladies* traces the long and complex history that has unfolded over the past 150 years between women, alcohol, their doctors, their families, and those concerned with women's social roles and health. Making strong use of archival materials and popular culture, McClellan shows how "alcoholics" (a term that came into widespread use in the early decades of the twentieth century, replacing the earlier preferred term "inebriate") came to include women, and how the female drinker complicated conventional narratives about intoxication and gender identity as she transformed from a "fallen angel" in the late nineteenth century into the "lit lady" of the 1950s. As McClellan effectively shows, a century and a half of women drinking have transformed the way Americans view alcohol and social relations, illuminating the "deeply gendered boundaries between acceptable and unacceptable use, between medicinal and recreational consumption, and between commercialized, public venues and private, domestic space" (p. 11).

McClellan moves chronologically, from the late nineteenth century into the twenty-first, showing how women's alcohol use has always posed a problem. Excessive drinking, especially by working-class prostitutes and immigrants, was seen as particularly debased in the late 1800s, and an action taken only by those who existed outside the bounds of "true" womanhood. Meanwhile, middle-class women—many of whom were on the side of temperance—were viewed as morally upright, respectable, and, most of all, sober. As the movement for Prohibition gained steam, women were seen as protectors of the family home, and they opposed their husbands' use of the saloon because alcohol drained financial resources, caused behavioral problems, and ruined the safety and security of the family realm. Women who participated in saloon life were seen as contributing to the problem, and in doing so, further destroying conventional family life.

But women did drink in the nineteenth century, as McClellan shows. Some women used alcohol as a medicine to relieve generalized "female complaints," which often stemmed from difficult childbirths. McClellan tells the

Nursing History Review 28 (2020): 215–217. A Publication of the American Association for the History of Nursing. Copyright © 2020 Springer Publishing Company.
http://dx.doi.org/10.1891/1062-8061.28.215

story of "Mrs. C.," a 25-year-old mother of two who was prescribed wine by her doctor to assist with pain after a prolonged labor, but who quickly turned to whiskey and brandy as her cravings increased. This form of iatrogenic addiction was a problem, McClellan argues, because drinking women were insufficient mothers—irritable, abusive, dismissive, and cold, they were the opposite of the warm and loving caretakers women were expected to be. Since childbearing and rearing were considered women's most important roles, the "fallen angels" who transformed into "inebriates" were pitiable creatures, worthier of sympathy than denigration, but still a problem. Doctors worried that women were more difficult to treat than men, and that their drinking would have unintended effects on that most important social sphere: the family.

These fears didn't lighten as America moved toward Prohibition. The eighteenth Amendment pushed drinking underground, and women into the speakeasy. As women drank alongside men, they disrupted traditional demarcations between the social spheres and the sexes. The "new woman" demanded the right to intoxication alongside her right to vote, work, and bob her hair. Meanwhile, "lit ladies," who drank at home, continued to pose a problem. It was assumed that women didn't know "how" to drink, and when they did, they became unmanageable. Looking for a release from the "burdens" of domestic duties, doctors believed that women's drinking sought to put women on equal footing with men—a dangerous and pathological goal.

McClellan spends most of her book analyzing the mid-century, focusing on the story of Margaret "Marty" Mann, who admitted her own alcoholism in a 1963 story in *Reader's Digest*. Mann was the first female member of Alcoholics Anonymous, and she spent her life trying to ensure that female alcoholics were treated under the same "disease paradigm" that slowly began to reign in the field of men's alcoholism studies. Arguing that women had "more to overcome than men," McClellan reveals how women seeking treatment for alcohol had to deal with prejudiced doctors, sexist AA members, and a medical establishment that didn't recognize their issue as a medical problem. Women's drinking was consistently seen as a symptom of the failure to "adjust" to conventional roles, even as men's drinking was seen as a chronic disease, and female drunks were seen as "especially debased." McClellan uses several notable resources here, including first-person narratives and a close reading of the 1962 film *Days of Wine and Roses*, to effectively prove her point.

Showing how women have always complicated the medicalization of alcoholism as a disease, McClellan provides useful new insights into the history of American alcohol use. But the book cuts off abruptly in mid-century, with McClellan waiting until the epilogue to offer a rather rushed reading of women and alcohol from Betty Ford to today. Still, by placing women back into the history of how alcoholism was defined and treated over the past 150 years, and by proving how women consistently muddied those waters, *Lady Lushes* is an intelligent and thorough examination of alcohol, medicine, and gender over the past two centuries.

EMILY DUFTON, PHD
TAKOMA PARK, MD

Fixing the Poor: Eugenic Sterilization and Child Welfare in the Twentieth Century

By Molly Ladd-Taylor

(Baltimore, MD: Johns Hopkins University Press, 2017) (304 pages; $54.95 hardcover)

In her intriguing new book, *Fixing the Poor: Eugenic Sterilization and Child Welfare in the Twentieth Century*, Molly Ladd-Taylor deftly draws upon fresh archival evidence on sterilization, institutionalization, eugenics, and understandings of delinquency and disability and in doing so, amends our understanding of the origins and purpose of the welfare state. Rather than framing sterilization as a product of a eugenics-obsessed state focused on the ultimate goal of "race betterment," she instead places the procedure and its goals within a "broad set of social welfare polices" aimed at reducing dependency and the "problems of poverty, sex, and single motherhood" (p. 2). In doing so, she moves the ongoing scholarship around the history of both welfare and eugenic policy away from simplistic binaries, and illustrates the ways they together "reflected and reworked popular and scientific ideas about race, gender, disability, and modernity itself" (p. 4).

The book teases out three broad themes over the course of six chapters—sterilization's key place in the contributing to the development of the emerging child welfare system of the era, sterilization's relationship with institutionalization, and how the all-encompassing concept of "feeblemindedness" was "used to justify both segregation and sterilization" (p. 3). Ladd-Taylor's evidence is rooted in the records of the state of Minnesota which featured a less restrictive program of sterilization and confinement than other states, and the program's "unremarkable quality[ies]" there also help to "expand our understanding of the spectrum of sterilization programs." Rather than targeting people of color for sterilization as in other states like California and North Carolina, Minnesota instead focused its efforts on those it deemed delinquent and dependent —unmarried mothers, "sex delinquents" and the general "dependent poor."

Yet, as Ladd-Taylor notes, the implementation of Minnesota welfare and eugenic policy was inconsistent and shaped by a variety of stakeholders. Authorities often disagreed on the nature of the linkages between feeblemindedness and delinquency, and many emphasized close community surveillance as a long-term solution rather than permanent institutionalization. As

Nursing History Review 28 (2020): 218–220. A Publication of the American Association for the History of Nursing. Copyright © 2020 Springer Publishing Company.
http://dx.doi.org/10.1891/1062-8061.28.218

Ladd-Taylor puts it, "More and more, experts distinguished between innocent feeble-minded people who could live under supervision . . . and defective delinquents who would always remain a menace" (p. 68).

One of the book's particularly striking points here centers on the gender gap between the two sentiments and how this gap complicated the full picture of both welfare and sterilization. Female social workers and supporters of maternalist women's clubs often advocated for "humanitarian" programs such as work colonies or halfway houses that helped feebleminded women find jobs and live in a supervised, safe environment. The Minnesota State Board of Control (a three-person panel appointed by the governor that functioned as the guardian for each "feebleminded" ward of the state) noted in 1924, "It will never be possible to herd all defectives into institutions and their useful labor under supervision will be an economic gain to the community" (p. 71). Echoing these same ideas, the Women's Welfare League noted for their records the benefit to sending "feebleminded girls . . . back into social life, under supervision, making them self-supporting and happy" (p. 71).

Of course, as Ladd-Taylor astutely notes, both community surveillance and institutional segregation were two sides of the same policy, but nevertheless these more expansive views of the capacities of the feebleminded clashed sharply with many hardline male eugenicists. Men such as Charles Fremont Dight, founder of the Minnesota Eugenics Society, "disdained the welfare-oriented eugenics that the Board of Control and most Minnesota reformers espoused . . . [and] had harsh words for maternalists . . ." Dight argued that no amount of "medical, surgical, or hospital care, prayers, tears, or repentance" could undo "bad heredity" (p. 78). He and a few other prominent men supported a sweeping sterilization law that had the authority to put anyone who was "obviously unfit" under the knife. Yet Dight and his supporters were rebuffed in their quest to widen the law to its utmost capacity by a variety of reformers, who instead advocated a broad set of measures to prevent, control, and reduce both "bad blood" and "bad behavior." These disagreements, often gendered, thus ultimately resulted in comprehensive yet inconsistently applied policies. The one constant, as Ladd-Taylor argues was the emphasis on incorporating eugenic policy as a tool of broader welfare initiatives aimed at reducing "the burden on the public purse" (p. 29). Sterilization would, as the book's title suggests, literally "fix" the poor physically, as well as financially.

Fixing the Poor's minute detailing of state politics and novel framing of the relationship between eugenics and welfare in Minnesota necessarily raises questions about how its arguments might apply in other case studies of other states. But its careful research also makes it an excellent addition to the wider canon of scholarship on the eugenics movement in the United States and the broader Progressive Era. Those interested in the histories of medicine, social work, state and local policy, and public health will find a wealth of new points to consider here.

LAUREN MACIVOR THOMPSON
Georgia State University

Building Resistance: Children, Tuberculosis, and the Toronto Sanatorium

By Stacy Burke

(Chicago, IL: McGill-Queen's University Press, 2018) (576 pages; $120.00 hardcover; $39.95 paperback; $39.95 electronic)

Stacy Burke's *Building Resistance* is a qualitative case study using historical data that explores the experiences of children hospitalized in the Toronto sanatorium with a focus on the time period between 1900 and 1950. Her time period begins with the initial years of sanatoriums across Canada and ends with the rise of antibiotics as a common treatment for tuberculosis. Her qualitative case study includes a vast sample of patient charts to mine richly descriptive themes as she fleshes out the children's lived experiences.

Burke references medical records, notes found in patient files, and an understanding of common medical and hospital practices in sanatoriums of the time period. Burke outlines adaptability, tuberculosis genealogies, resistance building, and responsibility as key organizational themes found in the data. The most broad and fascinating of these, resistance building, flows throughout her work as a dominant theme both in the lived experience as well as in the medical approaches to treatment.

Building Resistance stands at the intersection of the history of children's healthcare during the first half of the twentieth century, the social history of tuberculosis during her time period, and the focus on seeking patients' lived experiences with disease. This work describes each child's lived experience with illness. Used together with social histories, such as Barbara Bates work *Bargaining for Life*, Burke's insight into the world of Toronto sanatorium's young patients has great potential to broaden our critical thinking about this illness during the first half of the twentieth century.

Burke introduces her readers to children with intense detail. Their families, preferences, and day-to-day activities permeate her chapters and augment the thematic organization and underpinning. She masterfully incorporates personal letters written by family members as well as the children, photographs, and patients' oral histories highlighting both unique experiences as well as broader shared experiences. Burke creatively includes a chapter focused on the children's conduct sheets and report cards during their sanatorium stay.

Nursing History Review 28 (2020): 221–222. A Publication of the American Association for the History of Nursing. Copyright © 2020 Springer Publishing Company.
http://dx.doi.org/10.1891/1062-8061.28.221

While she admits this data relates most consistently to the children's misconduct and not particularly to their medical care, she draws from non-medical records such as notes passed in class between friends to explore how these children used their agency in the experiences of sometimes long and grueling separation from family and home.

Burke outlines the focus and need for its theoretical underpinning, it fails to thoroughly analyze its data. While she uses her qualitative training to explore the data and draw out masterful nuances in understanding how life played out for these children, she fails to treat her data for what it is: historical. She admittedly holds time as a constant despite the vast changes that occurred during her time period encompassing the First World War, the Great Depression, and the Second World War. Her data cannot be divorced from the social and cultural contexts that had deep influences on medical treatments, changing views on children and their value to society and family life, as well as family values and the ways families coped with death and disease. These themes must be understood within their own context. Thorough analytic consideration must be founded on the reality of change over time particularly if that time is different than our own.

While she teases out the children as unique patients, her work never proves the importance of why children's experiences and stories need to be a focal point. Burke herself briefly highlights that tuberculosis and diseases like it are making a comeback globally in our current time and are not strictly diseases of the past, but she fails to elaborate on why the need for her work is critical today. *Building Resistance* has great potential to inform our understanding of the challenges faced by children and families who face chronic illnesses today with a more critical understanding of her data's rich historical context.

While Burke's work would be enriched by a skillful blending of qualitative and historical methodologies, I recommend this work to students and scholars interested in exploring the lived experiences of children and healthcare, tuberculosis as a widespread disease, and the development of sanatoriums in Canada in the early twentieth century. Her data and creative lens are an asset to thinking critically about this topic and might enable us to ask more nuanced questions about illness, children's unique perspectives, and our own ability to resist immense and seemingly insurmountable challenges.

BRIANA RALSTON SMITH
Children's Hospital of Philadelphia
Philadelphia, PA

Living With Lead: An Environmental History of Idaho's Coeur D'Alenes, 1885–2011

By Bradley D. Snow

(Pittsburgh, PA: University of Pittsburgh Press, 2017) (275 pages; $28.95 paper)

The population of Kellogg, Idaho never exceeded 6,000. It is a small town with a huge toxic legacy. For almost a century, the mines and smelters around Kellogg produced tens of billions of dollars worth of silver, zinc, and lead. The land holding the ore, the workers who disgorged and transformed it, and the citizens in the smelters' shadow all bore the brunt of that fateful alchemy.

Most modern historical scholarship on lead and lead poisoning focuses on the human health costs of lead in consumer goods, whether paint, gasoline, or the water pipes in our homes delivering hot and cold running poison. A significant thread examines lead poisoning in occupational settings. Bradley Snow's *Living with Lead* turns the focus to the other end of the lead economy. Unlike the settings for most lead poisoning histories—New York, Baltimore, Chicago—Kellogg's toxic exposures came not from consumption but production of metals, both precious silver and the baser but "useful metal" lead.

Snow opens with a chapter on the history of Kellogg itself. The legend of gold prospector Noah Kellogg wandering the Idaho countryside in 1885, and how his four-legged companion led him to a rich outcropping of galena ore, quickly turns to another familiar tale of the West: the rise of the highly capitalized large-scale industrial operations it takes to extract silver, zinc, and lead from that galena ore. Directly in the shadows of those operations rose a prosperous company town. The chapter ends with the town of Kellogg many decades later, after those mines and smelters were shuttered, a post-industrial community groping for a future.

After a brief survey of the history of lead poisoning from ancient days to the end of the twentieth century, the book's central four chapters examine four distinct paths of harm Kellogg's mining and smelting followed: through rivers, the atmosphere, the bodies of the regions inhabitants, and the workers inside the plants. Snow first examines mining's death-dealing impact on the Coeur d'Alene River—the natural consequence of the world view of an industry that, in Snow's droll understatement, "did not, as a rule, put much thought or energy into questions involving the ecological impact of their operations" (p. 85). From waterways choked by mine tailings, Snow moves to the

Nursing History Review 28 (2020): 223–225. A Publication of the American Association for the History of Nursing. Copyright © 2020 Springer Publishing Company.
http://dx.doi.org/10.1891/1062-8061.28.223

output of the smelters, which for decades spewed sulfur dioxide, arsenic, cadmium, and lead into the air, turning forest and farmland into acidic dead zones. Chapter 5 turns to the public health impact of this airborne environmental assault. In a variation on a familiar story, an industrial accident in 1973 sends an abnormal bolus of fine lead particulates into Kellogg's skies, spiking residents' blood lead levels, and prompting a long-overdue reckoning with the chronic exposures that had been sickening the town's citizens all along. The statistics shock even the historian familiar with the norms of lead in mid-century America: in 1975, *average* blood leads in children living between 1 and 2.5 miles of the Bunker Hill Company's smelter hovered near 60µg/dL. Then CDC director William Foege labeled the region "the site of the worst community lead exposure problem in the United States" (p. 135). Turning to the scene behind the factory doors, Chapter 6 discusses those who had been "on Lead's Front Lines" from the start—the mine and smelter workers. Their story too is familiar in occupational health history: poisoned by the only job in town, their desires for a safe work environment often took a back seat to bread-and-butter issues. Early on, Kellogg's lead factories fell under the scrutiny of federal health researchers, and with the advent of worker's compensation laws, they implemented measurable improvements in hygiene and safety conditions. But improvements in Kellogg's factories tended to lag behind those in large industrial cities.

These four chapters are arranged thematically, not chronologically, each chapter following its subject from decades ago to efforts in recent years to redeem the land, cleanse the waters, or lower the burden of lead exposure in workers and children. Thus, we see the despoliation, nearly overnight, of the Coeur d'Alene a century ago, the mining companies' belated and insufficient improvements in containing tailings in the early 1960s, their battles with the newly-minted Environmental Protection Agency [EPA] in the 1970s, and the mixed success after the smelters shut down in the early 1980s, at restoring aquatic plant and animal life to stretches of the river. The chapter on community health ends with the abatement of lead-saturated topsoil and house dust, a herculean effort that brought Kellogg's average blood lead levels in line with typical urban environments nationwide. Chapter 6 ends with workers fighting for their jobs, even signaling their willingness to accept deadly compromises in safety requirements in order to keep the smelters—their only viable shot at a stable income for their families—from shuttering permanently.

But close they did, and the last substantive chapter tells of the Kellogg region's efforts to reinvent itself as a tourist destination, a Bavarian ski village replete with "Willkommen zu Kellogg" signs and North America's longest gondola. "Once a strong union town filled with home owning hard hats and busy merchants," Snow observes, "Kellogg's shrunken population now struggles to sell lattes and condos to out-of-state visitors" (p. 11). Ironically, the largest economic force in the area over the last generation has been the EPA. The massive cleanup of Superfund sites in the region brought hundreds of long-term jobs, with locals filling the vast majority of positions.

Living With Lead originated as a Ph.D. dissertation, and despite its generally engaging narrative voice and engaging structure, its academic roots show through here and there, most notably in the occasional tangents into theoretical or historiographical backroads. But the book's heart is the rich research Snow conducted in local, government, and industry sources. It will be useful for scholars looking to fill gaps in the historiography of lead poisoning, or educators looking for compelling examples from that history. It provides a biography of sorts of a unique region and its people, and, always in the background, America in its tragic century of lead.

CHRISTIAN WARREN
Brooklyn College
Department of History

Historia de la Enfermería: Evolución Histórica del Cuidado Enfermero, Third Edition History of Nursing: Historical Evolution of Nursing Care, Third Edition

By María Luisa Martínez and Elena Chamorro Rebollo

(Barcelona, Spain: Elsevier, 2017) (188 pages; $25.00 paperback)

Generations of nurses have learned little history in college and will learn none throughout their career. This is a constant grievance among faculty nurses in Spanish-speaking circles. Things seem to be changing, however. Martínez and Chamorro are the authors, most recently, of one of the most widely available nursing history books in contemporary Spain. This is the third edition of a 2007 book authored by Martín and Martínez. We are warned that this is a book primarily aimed at nursing students and practicing nurses, and we soon learn why.

The opening chapter situates the reader in a common ground: styles of nursing care that coincide roughly with "stages" of the development of nursing as an occupation. They begin with ancient civilizations (domestic nursing) to move forward in phases through to the contemporary age (professional nursing). In so doing, the authors use as a blueprint a view that owes much to Collière's[1] linear pattern of development, which has been enormously influential in Spain as well as in Latin America.

Chapter 1 somewhat elaborates on the first phase, and understandably, it offers little more than a speculative narrative of how the care of the sick might have been during pre-history and the antiquity. This chapter, nonetheless, gives us an interesting glossary of terms, each worth exploring in depth.

Chapter 2 covers what here is called "the vocational phase" of care, which ranges from the rise of Christianity to the Middle Ages to the Pre-Modern Era. The reader will note an unmistakable focus on religious orders, over relying perhaps on stories of manuals written by monastic nurses to describe their deed. Although the seasoned nursing historian may faint to see how quickly we are taken through centuries of history in some thirty pages, one is at least pleased to see an acknowledgment to something unique to Spanish nursing: its close contact with the Islamic world. As recognized, the ethnocentric term Middle Ages is used to refer pejoratively to a period of European history, while other cultures flourished around the same era acting as reservoirs of knowledge during the great intellectual oppression in Europe. The Arabs preserved

Nursing History Review 28 (2020): 226–228. A Publication of the American Association for the History of Nursing. Copyright © 2020 Springer Publishing Company.
http://dx.doi.org/10.1891/1062-8061.28.226

manuscripts in Latin and Greek that were later translated from Arabic into European languages. In a way, the essence of this pivotal process is captured in this chapter, which is often neglected in histories of science and health.

The beginning of the Late Modern period (*Edad Contemporánea*) is traced back in Chapter 3 to the French Revolution. To this era, other turning points are loosely attributed, including the rise of capitalism as a system upon which industrial relations are based. Expectedly, a great deal of space is devoted to Nightingale's prouesse. However, there is no linkage between the armed conflict for world domination with the events being recalled, which obscures the participation of non-English nurses and underscores one ethnocentric view on history that has been passed on by the oral tradition during a century and a half. The rest of the chapter is a well-known story of scientific discoveries and formalization of professions.

By the second half of the book, these phases are still treated as *the* model of history. Although a sequence of stages is a frame that the target readership will immediately recognize and feel familiar with, an acknowledgment to the limitations of Whiggish history would not have gone astray.

Focusing on nursing as a distinct system of knowledge, Chapter 4 brings together interesting pieces of the global history and the European system of education, coupled with the interests of supranational organizations as far as health is concerned. This part, however, is more disciplinary than it is historical.

Chapter 5, the novelty of the present edition, addresses ongoing processes of change in Spain. While the "history of the present" normally implies that contemporary events are reconstructed and looked at with a historical gaze, a link between past and present is simply missing here. We are given an account of professional affairs largely using institutional landmarks as the navigation device for the profession. It would have been insightful, and indeed customary for a book of this type, to see how decisions about new challenges may be informed by history. But we are left wondering why this did not happen.

Other histories of nursing and midwifery have been published in Spanish meanwhile. Two excellent examples are Biernat, Cerdá and Ramacciotti's[2] in Argentina, and Zárate's[3] in Chile, which have been crafted to perfection on the basis of meticulous archival research—the one drawing attention to the participation of nurses in contemporary history, and the other illustrating the appropriation of pregnancy and birth by scientific medicine. Necessarily, these are devoted to narrower periods of history.

Efforts to revitalise nursing history in the Spanish-speaking world must be celebrated. And this one offers a myriad of interesting ideas. Yet, as its predecessors, the 2017 edition of Martínez and Chamorro's suffers from serious methodological flaws, and for the same reason its overarching title promises something impossible.

Notes

1. M. F. Collière, *Promover la Vida [Promoting Life]* (Madrid, Spain: McGraw-Hill, 1993).

2. C. Bierna, J. M. Cerdá and K. I. Ramacciotti, *La Salud Pública y la Enfermería en la Argentina [Public Health and Nursing in Argentina]* (Buenos Aires, Argentina: Universidad Nacional de Quilmes, 2015).

3. M. S. Zárate, *Dar a Luz en Chile: De la "Ciencia de Hembra" a la Ciencia Obstétrica [Giving Birth in Chile: From Female Science to Obstetric Science]* (Santiago, Chile: Ediciones Universidad Alberto Hurtado, 2007).

RICARDO A. AYALA
Department of Sociology
Ghent University
Belgium

On the Other Hand: Left Hand, Right Brain, Mental
Disorder, and History
By Howard I. Kushner
(Baltimore, MD: Johns Hopkins Press, 2017) (200 pages; $26.95 hardcover)

This book is about a problem that is not really a problem. In *On the Other Hand,* noted historian of science and medicine Howard Kushner tracks a century or more of studies into left-handedness, laterality, and brain asymmetry. His conclusion: that there is no concrete verifiable evidence that left-handedness is a problem. For most readers in North America or Western Europe, this might come as no surprise. Gone are the days when left-handed students are forced to switch hands. But as Kushner demonstrates, for over a century, scientists from a range of disciplines have tried to understand the cause and effects of left-handedness (and laterality more generally), often assuming that left-handedness is either specifically pathological or a proxy for some other form of disability. *On the Other Hand* traces this history, linking scientific discipline with paradigms and methods, tracking the rise and fall of cultural explanations and the growing dominance of genetics. Ultimately, Kushner argues that the assumption that left-handedness is abnormal lies in deep-seated beliefs about the sacred and the profane, a set of beliefs to which a century or more of research has added a patina of science. And while this research has, in turn, prompted intriguing questions about brain asymmetry, laterality and language acquisition, the fact that left-handedness is, indeed, quite normal (affecting somewhere between 5% and 25% of the population), remains. So what has all the fuss (and research) been about?

Over time, researchers have connected left-handedness with criminality, with primitivism, with arrested psychological development, learning disabilities, autism, schizophrenia, sexual preference, and occasionally, with creative talent and superior intelligence. And so it was these other subjects that studies in handedness were meant to illuminate.

And yet scientists have struggled to find a consistent and workable definition of handedness. By the mid-twentieth century two relatively short survey-based inventories came to dominate handedness testing: the Annett and the Oldfield inventories. Moving beyond writing and drawing (the common indicators used by teachers) the Annett and Oldfield inventories asked about a

Nursing History Review 28 (2020): 229–231. A Publication of the American Association for the History of Nursing. Copyright © 2020 Springer Publishing Company.
http://dx.doi.org/10.1891/1062-8061.28.229

range of activities, in order to understand better how handedness might exist along a continuum. Still questions about the reliability of such tests remain. In societies where left-handedness is stigmatized, would people feel free to answer honestly? Indeed, it would seem they do not as the numbers are lowest in those places (China and India, for example) where considerable effort is made to switch left-handed students to use their right hands and highest in places where such practices have faded (Western Europe and North America). Additionally, how would someone who has switched hands for some tasks answer the questions? If this sort of definitional imprecision is not enough, recently scientists have come to use the term "non-right-handed" as a more capacious category with which to work.

Trying to find the cause of laterality and its effects has embroiled scientists in classic nature vs. nurture debates. The most famous environmental explanation was that of Norman Geschwind and colleagues Peter Behan and Albert Galaburda who argued that stress during pregnancy caused elevated testosterone levels which damaged the left hemisphere. This helped explain the fact that there were more male than female left-handers while also suggesting that testosterone interfered with the maturation of the thymus leading to autoimmune disorders. But when they tried to verify their hypothesis using large population-based studies, left-handedness turned out to be an unreliable predictor of other disorders.

Meanwhile genetic research came to dominate the scientific landscape in the later twentieth century, and studies of handedness were no exception. The heritability of handedness was well known but scientists debated whether the mechanism was the disruption of the dominant gene for right-handedness or the inheritance of a recessive left-handed gene or, more recently, the effect of a combination of genetic and epigenetic factors. Thinking genetically about handedness has also opened the door to more trans-species research questioning the assumption that laterality is a uniquely human characteristic. If not, as some of these studies indicate, studying laterality in animals raises intriguing questions about language acquisition through evolution.

As historical work, *On the Other Hand,* handles well how dominant paradigms have changed over time and how research networks and funding contribute to what questions are asked and the methods used to answer them. But Kushner does a much better job situating handedness research in the social, cultural, and political contexts of the early twentieth century than he does that latter part of the century. We are left wondering what the persistence of handedness research suggests about our own times and what the shift to genetic explanations from environmental ones means for us. Still *On the*

Other Hand, offers a deft interweaving of the various disciplines—sciences and social sciences—that have studied handedness and the larger questions they sought to answer through such work.

Mary-Ellen Kelm
Simon Fraser University
Burnaby, British Columbia
Canada

Imperfect Pregnancies: A History of Birth Defects and
Prenatal Diagnosis

By Ilana Löwy

(Baltimore, MD: Johns Hopkins University Press, 2017) (277 pages; $44.95
hardcover)

In *Imperfect Pregnancies: A History of Birth Defects and Prenatal Diagnosis*, historian of science Ilana Löwy relates the complicated history of the development of prenatal testing of the fetus, from precursor science in the nineteenth century to the present. Löwy's approach is ambitious, because as she notes, this history can only be properly understood through an examination of the entire prenatal diagnosis *dispositif* (often translated as "apparatus" in English versions of Michel Foucault's writings). Löwy aims to explain not just the science, but also the social, political, medical, bureaucratic, and industrial contributions to the way prenatal diagnosis has been developed and integrated into routine prenatal care. Löwy follows these historical developments as they unfold internationally, primarily in the European and American countries in which the science was originally developed, but also briefly visiting Brazil and Japan. This sprawling history could have used a few more writerly signposts to organize the arguments, but an interested reader will find a great deal of informative analysis as well as a mature and nuanced perspective on a fraught topic.

Löwy tells a story of prenatal fetal surveillance that began with relatively limited testing in narrowly-defined groups of pregnant women considered at high risk for having a child with a birth defect, and eventually expanded into broad-scope screening tests that are offered to all pregnant woman as a routine part of prenatal care. She begins with a chapter explaining the nineteenth and early twentieth century rise of scientific and medical interest in understanding the causes of what had previously been labeled "monstrous" births, and in offering medical care before and during pregnancy which might prevent birth defects. Löwy next explains the scientific development of an understanding of chromosomes that underlay the initial introduction of amniocentesis in the 1960s and 1970s. Amniocentesis, an invasive test in which amniotic fluid is withdrawn via needle during the second trimester, was promoted in the 1970s as a way to test for conditions that are the result of extra or missing chromosomes (primarily Down Syndrome) as well as hereditary metabolic diseases.

Nursing History Review 28 (2020): 232–234. A Publication of the American Association for the History of Nursing. Copyright © 2020 Springer Publishing Company.
http://dx.doi.org/10.1891/1062-8061.28.232

It was offered to women who knew they carried these rare hereditary conditions, and to women over the age of 40, who were at highest risk of having a fetus with Down Syndrome.

Coinciding with the scientific and technological know-how to offer amniocentesis was the legalization of abortion across much of the West. As much as abortion was offered as a "solution" to birth defects, all involved understood that it was not the same as a cure. Political debates and personal dilemmas around abortion are a theme throughout the history Löwy relates, continuing up to the present, and they have been a constant, if sometimes submerged, undercurrent to public discussion.

Developments in the lab and the clinic broadened the scope of prenatal testing. By the early 1990s, a combination of ultrasound imaging and blood tests could be used to screen for Down Syndrome, and in some countries was offered routinely to pregnant women, whether at high or low risk for birth defects. This was non-invasive testing that did not put a pregnancy at risk of miscarriage (as amniocentesis did). If a woman tested positive, she was referred for amniocentesis. In a low-risk population, the vast majority of positive screens were false positives. The side-effects of screening—weeks of agonizing worry and a risk of miscarriage of a healthy fetus—impacted many otherwise uncomplicated pregnancies.

False positive screening results were not the only problematic side effect of prenatal screening. Löwy spends a chapter describing the dilemmas around incidental diagnoses of extra or missing sex chromosomes, which produce relatively mild syndromes. Should these differences in chromosomes be considered "defects" indicating therapeutic abortion? In the last few years, recently-developed tests which compare cell-free DNA in maternal blood to a "normal" DNA template have been commercialized and marketed aggressively. They provide much data, but not necessarily clarity. What should be done when a genetic anomaly not linked to a known birth defect is identified, as often happens? How are parent–child relationships impacted by test results that suggest something may be wrong, but do not provide a clear diagnosis?

Löwy urges her reader to attend to the dilemmas and difficulties caused by the proliferation and normalization of prenatal testing. She argues that too much of our focus has been on slippery slope arguments about eugenics and "designer babies," when the more mundane but equally worrisome problems caused by ubiquitous screening have sneaked in right under our noses, in the guise of incremental improvements to routine and accepted prenatal care. Parents, she persuasively argues, are not seeking perfect children; rather, they are seeking perfect assurance that their children will not have devastating disabilities. Still, as the history of prenatal testing shows, that reassurance comes with a steep price. Knowing the history, we have a better chance to make a clear-eyed decision about whether we are willing to pay it.

LARA FREIDENFELDS, PhD
New Jersey

Cesarean Section: An American History of Risk, Technology, and Consequence

By Jacqueline H. Wolf

(Baltimore, MD: Johns Hopkins University Press, 2017) (320 pages; $49.95 hardcover)

Jacqueline Wolf's book on the rise of the cesarean section over the last century makes a strong argument: the increase in the cesarean rate is the result of a misguided shift in understandings of risk in childbirth. The causes she identifies are incremental, building in complexity over time and contributing eventually to a meteoric rise in c-sections during the 1970s and 1980s, and beyond. Today, she notes, the rate has reached alarming heights, peaking well over 30%, a number that far surpasses historical and global health evidence that identifies a "true" complication rate of just 5%–6% (pp. 4–5).

Over the course of seven well-researched and persuasively-written chapters, Wolf demonstrates how an operation that doctors once approached with universal dread became the routinized procedure it is today. Between the late nineteenth century and the first few decades of the twentieth, the rise of hospital maternity wards and the adoption of anesthesia, aseptic and antiseptic techniques, uterine sutures, and earlier medical intervention reduced the horror associated with the procedure in the previous era. By the end of the 1920s, she notes, doctors were able to approach the cesarean in a calmer, more planned manner that, when combined with improved surgical techniques, improved outcomes. Slowly, the cesarean became "shorn of its terrors" (pp. 46). From there, the introduction of blood transfusions and antibiotics after World War II helped stave off mortality from hemorrhage and postpartum infection. Additional technologies over time, particularly the Friedman curve (a statistical tool used to determine whether a labor was progressing "on time"), the Apgar score (and the pressure it placed on doctors to get "good scores") and Electrical Fetal Monitoring (EFM), all created new complexities that seemed to simultaneously minimize the risks of cesarean, while increasing the perceived risks of vaginal delivery. These risks were not all equal, of course, but the threat of malpractice suits which grew in the 1970s and 1980s alongside the introduction of the supposedly irrefutable material evidence recorded by EFM, made doctors calculate risk differently (pp. 165–166).

Nursing History Review 28 (2020): 235–237. A Publication of the American Association for the History of Nursing. Copyright © 2020 Springer Publishing Company.
http://dx.doi.org/10.1891/1062-8061.28.235

Lest the reader accuse Wolf of technological determinism, she also examines some of the cultural shifts behind the rising c-section rate. Both within and outside of medicine, acceptance of unknown risk in childbirth became increasingly unacceptable. The unknowns, unpredictability, and uncontrollability of a vaginal delivery loomed larger over time, exacerbated, ironically, by the increasing numbers of female doctors into obstetrics at the end of the twentieth century. Driven by their own experiences of childbirth, and a preference for medicalized interventions, Wolf argues that female obstetricians have been able to act with dual authority—that of the physician and of the mother (or potential mother; pp. 177–179).

There is much of value in this work and it is truly impressive for its scope and clarity of argument. Maternal healthcare practitioners, policy makers, and historians will find this a must-read. Because of its relevance to contemporary healthcare, Wolf's take on the implications of these historical narratives is likely to evoke strong reactions. For example, Wolf states outright that cesarean sections performed for "elective" or "non-medical" reasons are ethically unjustifiable (p. 207). She also calls for the collection of more concrete data and improved training protocols in obstetric residency programs.

Her significant contribution to the historiography is also likely to spark conversations among scholars. There are points where Wolf's forceful argument overpowers other possibilities, interpretations, and voices. Despite integrating mothers' birth narratives into her final two chapters, for example, the reader is left to wonder about mothers' agency, voices, reasoning, and experiences in earlier chapters, as well. This is a story in which change appears to be driven primarily by doctors and structural forces that exist beyond women's control. One notable exception to this is the story Wolf tells about the resignation of U.S. obstetricians in finally accepting the low-transverse cesarean over the traditional classic method (pp. 156–163). Although they were years behind their European counterparts, American physicians finally adopted this method with lower risk of uterine tears at least partially because mothers pushed for access to vaginal births after c-sections (or VBACs).

Despite the work's admirable breadth, the argument steers away from a deep analysis of how the cesarean section's rise intersects with the changes in expectations and experiences of motherhood that have arisen over the past century. How did definitions of acceptable risk change for mothers as the meaning of motherhood itself changed over time? How have the changing material realities of mothers' lives shaped the framing of risk in childbirth? As one of Wolf's interviewees, April, shares: "I was prepared to take the risks with my body. I was not, however, prepared to take risks for the baby" (pp. 176). Wolf convincingly shows us how April acted within a system of contingencies created over a century: an under-trained obstetrician constrained by legal pressures and her own experience of childbirth; a hospital environment driven by technological diagnostics and professional standards and norms; and a mother, haunted by a prior birth experience and her desire for a healthy baby. The reader is left to wonder, however, how April herself understood and evaluated the risks involved in that moment—and why. Uncontextualized beyond their birth experiences, the mothers in Wolf's book tell us little about how race, family, community, ideological beliefs, or socioeconomic status have shaped how risk materializes and is enacted at the maternal bedside. In providing this foundational narrative, however, Wolf's book will likely shape debates surrounding childbirth and cesarean sections for years to come.

Jessica L. Martucci
Research Fellow
Science History Institute
315 Chestnut Street
Philadelphia, PA 19106

Artificial Hearts: The Allure and Ambivalence of a Controversial Medical Technology

By Shelley McKellar

(Baltimore, MD: Johns Hopkins University Press, 2018) (376 pages; $54.95 hardcover)

In *Artificial Hearts: The Allure and Ambivalence of a Controversial Medical Technology*, Shelley McKellar explores the technological, political, and cultural history of the artificial heart from the 1950s through the 2000s. Many of the actors and events in this book will be well-known to readers. Unlike previous books featuring Willem Kolff, Michael DeBakey and Denton Cooley however, their discoveries, outsized personalities, and public feuds are not the center of the narrative.[1] McKellar's approach to the history of artificial hearts is to place the devices themselves at the center of the story. The engineering achievements of total artificial hearts (TAHs) and vascular assist devices (VADs) are set within the context of shifting support for the devices within the medical sphere, the government, and the media in response to the only partial success of research programs and experimental surgeries. McKellar's main argument is that the *desire* for an operational artificial heart rather than the actual functionality of the devices drove the invention and implementation of technologies including the Jarvik-7 and Akutsu III. The author dissects the conflicting definitions of success held by different stakeholders in experimental TAH surgeries which resulted in ambiguous support for continued development of heart replacement technologies. The book is organized in a roughly chronological series of case studies, each centered on a particular device, its application in experimental and often controversial surgeries and the response of surgical outcomes among clinicians, patients, families and the media.

Chapter 1 describes the foundation of artificial heart research in the 1950s through the 1960s, a time when Americans had fully embraced science and technology as the answer to society's problems, including the heart disease epidemic. Heart failure, a condition that occurs when heart muscle progressively loses its ability to pump blood due to damage from heart disease had little effective treatment during this era. Kolff, DeBakey, and others were entirely confident that the TAH would be a game-changing cure for heart failure once they met the device's engineering challenges. McKellar describes how this optimism led to the growth of TAH research programs despite many technical setbacks

Nursing History Review 28 (2020): 238–240. A Publication of the American Association for the History of Nursing. Copyright © 2020 Springer Publishing Company.
http://dx.doi.org/10.1891/1062-8061.28.238

and negative patient outcomes. In Chapter 2, McKellar explores the role of the media in shaping public and government support for human heart transplants and TAH research through the much publicized conflict between DeBakey and Denton Cooley regarding the first TAH placement in 1969. The accomplishments and failures of heart transplants in the 1960s as well as the press coverage of the feud shaped TAHs as a "complementary" rather than a "competing" cardiac replacement therapy and tempered the public's enthusiasm for these devices. The third chapter identifies themes of risk in medical technology through the history of atomic-powered artificial hearts (1967–1977). McKellar argues that while this technology showed real promise in meeting the powering challenges of cardiac assistive devices, the public found the risks of atomic powered hearts were too high led to the phasing out of this approach. Chapter 4 focuses on the Utah TAH/Jarvik-7 program during the 1980s, dramatic transplant surgeries and sensationally publicized cases of TAH recipient Barney Clark and others. While the clinical experiments were initially celebrated as successful cures for heart failure, the poor quality of life, and uncertainty faced by recipients led to disillusionment with the technological promise of TAH. The medical community, the media, and bioethicists, an emerging voice in healthcare during the 1980s began to question the role of TAH in treating heart failure. McKellar argues that a lack of consensus over what "success" meant in TAH among stakeholders led to ambiguity regarding the future of TAH research creating a more challenging environment in which to research/develop TAH after the 1980s. Chapters 5 and 6 focus on the history of VADs, technologies that support a failing heart left intact. McKellar argues that VADs researchers were more successful in navigating their devices through clinical trials, regulatory requirements, and the marketplace than TAH researchers due in part to the relative simplicity of VADs but primarily through partnerships with established medical device companies. The final chapter includes case studies of TAHs the early 2000s and the continued advancement of TAH technologies, still imperfect. McKellar concludes with a discussion of the legacy of the history of the devices on today's debates about permanent TAH given the shortage of donor hearts and America's continued technological optimism.

The public backlash to the 1969 Jarvik-7 surgery included criticism that the considerable resources poured into developing TAHs would have been better spent on heart disease prevention. In her discussion of this debate, McKellar raises the question: what if a device wasn't the answer to treating heart failure? Her focus on TAH technology does not give the author space to fully explore this idea. Questioning why non-device and perhaps non-surgical approaches to heart failure posed no real threat to TAH research programs would add support to McKellar's main argument.

A historian of medical technology and surgery, McKellar expertly weaves medical and technical information into her narrative, a skill critical to the reader's understanding of the socio-cultural history of these complex devices. The author's argument that a device that *functions* but doesn't really *work* as a cardiac replacement therapy cannot be labeled a success relies on her discussion of the failure of TAH teams to anticipate and manage the after-effects of placement or even consider patient-sided technical challenges such as the biocompatibility of TAHs. *Artificial Hearts* will be of interest to historians of health and technology as well as nurses and other clinicians who manage the patient side of new devices.

Notes

1. See for example: G. Wayne Miller, *King of Hearts: The True Story of the Maverick Who Pioneered Open Heart Surgery* (New York: Crown, 2010); and Mimi Swartz, *Ticker: The Quest to Create an Artificial Heart* (New York: Crown, 2018).

Amanda L. Mahoney
Chief Curator
Dittrick Medical History Center
Case Western Reserve University
Cleveland, OH 44106

NEW DISSERTATIONS

Compiled for the Nursing History Review by Jonathon Erlen, PhD, History of Medicine Librarian, Health Sciences Library System, and Assistant Professor, Graduate School of Public Health at the University of Pittsburgh, Pittsburgh, PA. These dissertations can be obtained through Proquest Dissertations.

Tara Dosumo Diener, A Hospital in situ: Maternity Nursing Practice in Freetown since 1892, 2016 PhD Dissertation, University of Michigan. (Publication Number: 10391563).

Laura Roe Madden, Riding the waves of change: Oral Histories from Students of Georgia Baptist Hospital School of Nursing during the 1970s, 2016 PhD Dissertation, Mercer University. (Publication Number: 10302005).

Kathleen M. Nishida, St. Luke's College of Nursing, Tokyo, Japan: The Intersections of an Episcopal Church Mission Project, Rockefeller Foundation Philanthropy, and the Development of Nursing in Japan, 1918-1941, 2016, PhD Dissertation, University of Pennsylvania. (Publication Number: 10191916).

Nursing History Review 28 (2020): 241–242. A Publication of the American Association for the History of Nursing. Copyright © 2020 Springer Publishing Company.
http://dx.doi.org/10.1891/1062-8061.28.241

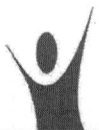

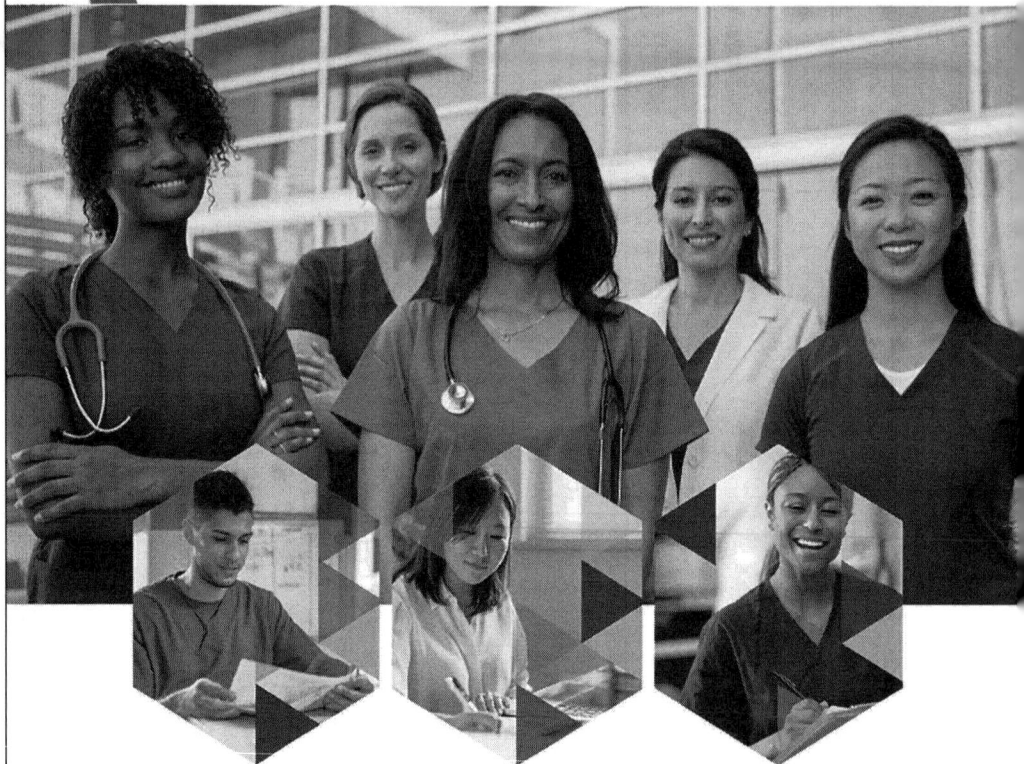